Coloring Book
for Adults
Relaxation and Reduce Stress

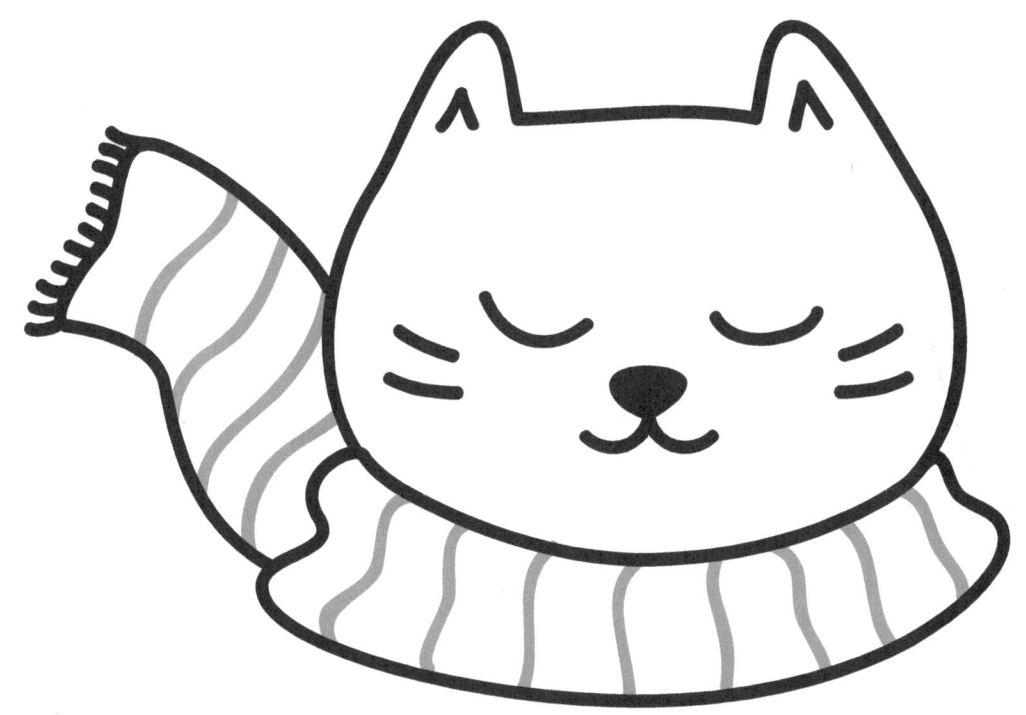

THIS COLORING

BOOK BELONGS TO

....

Coloring Book
by: Samuel Lyons

Check out my other products on Amazon, prepared for children and adults. I would also appreciate your opinion on this product on Amazon. Greetings and invite you inside!

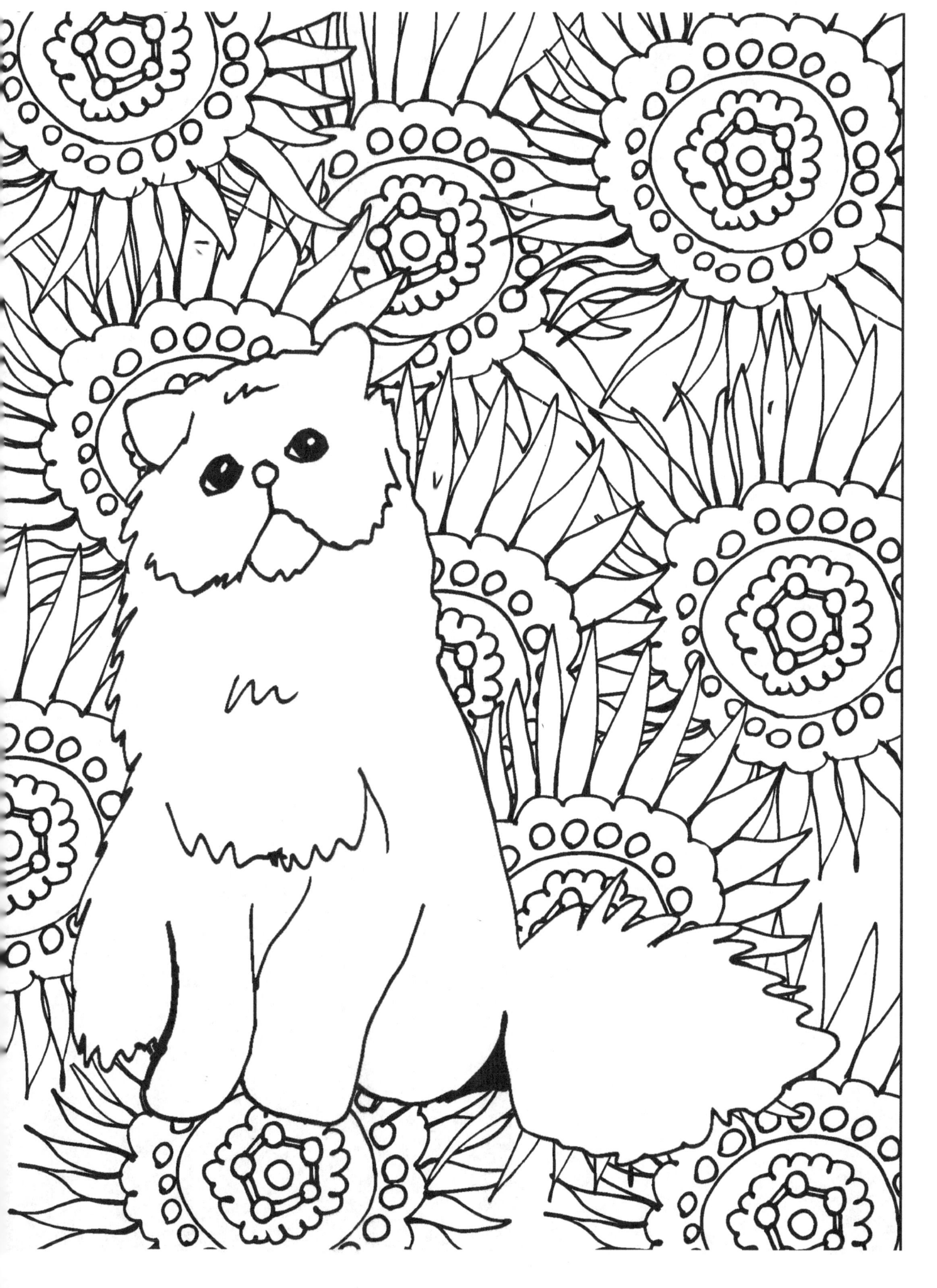

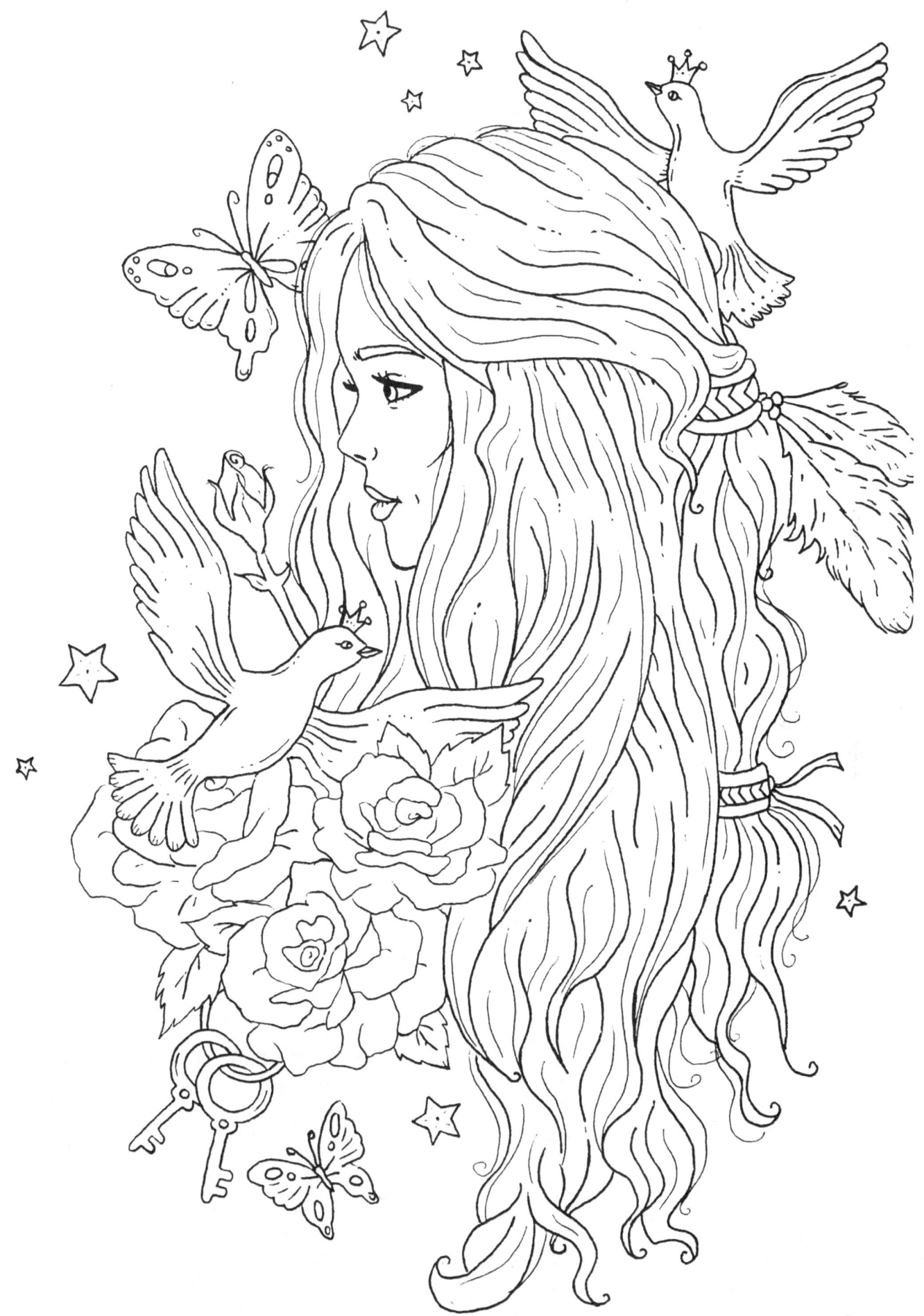

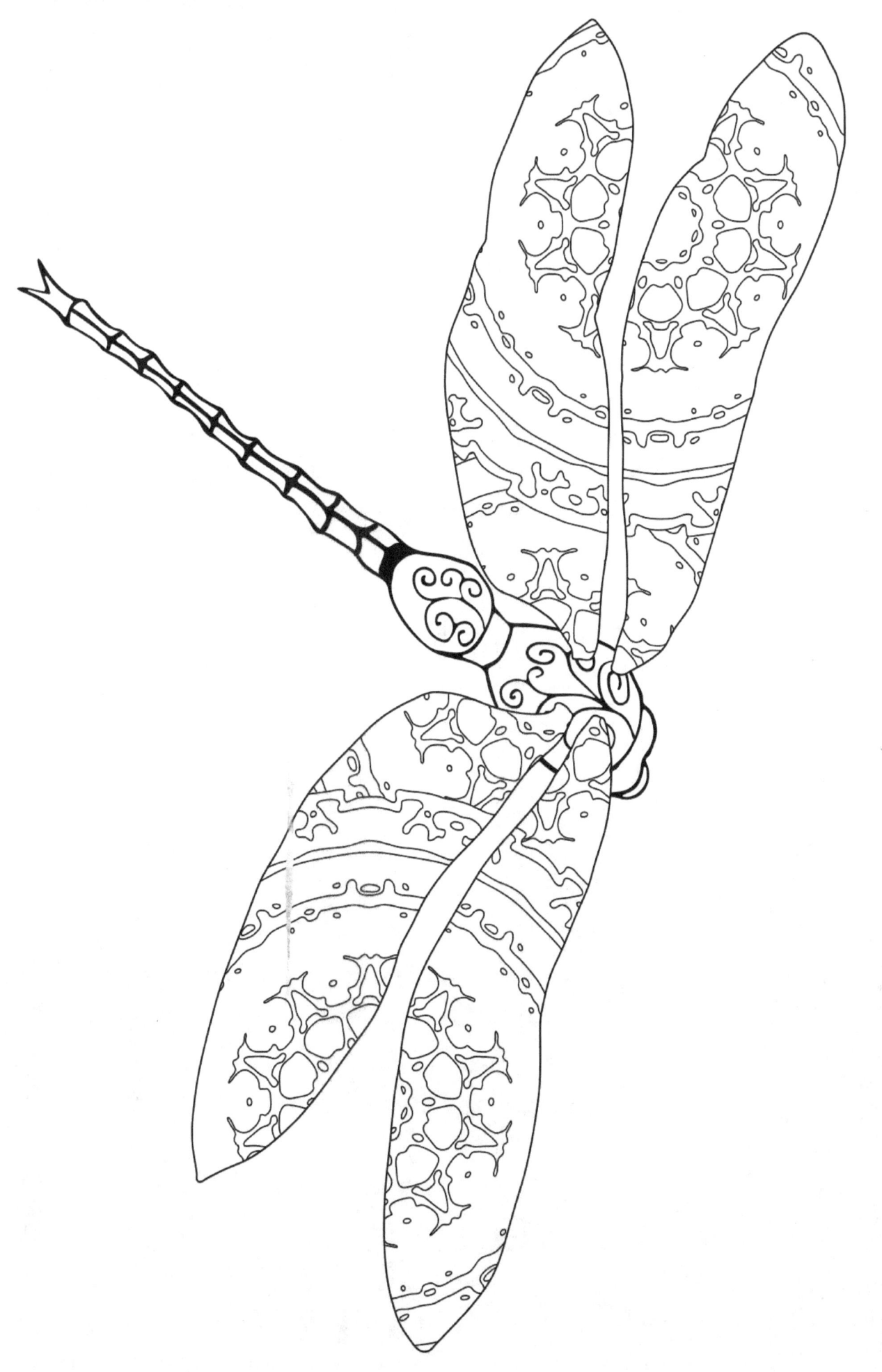

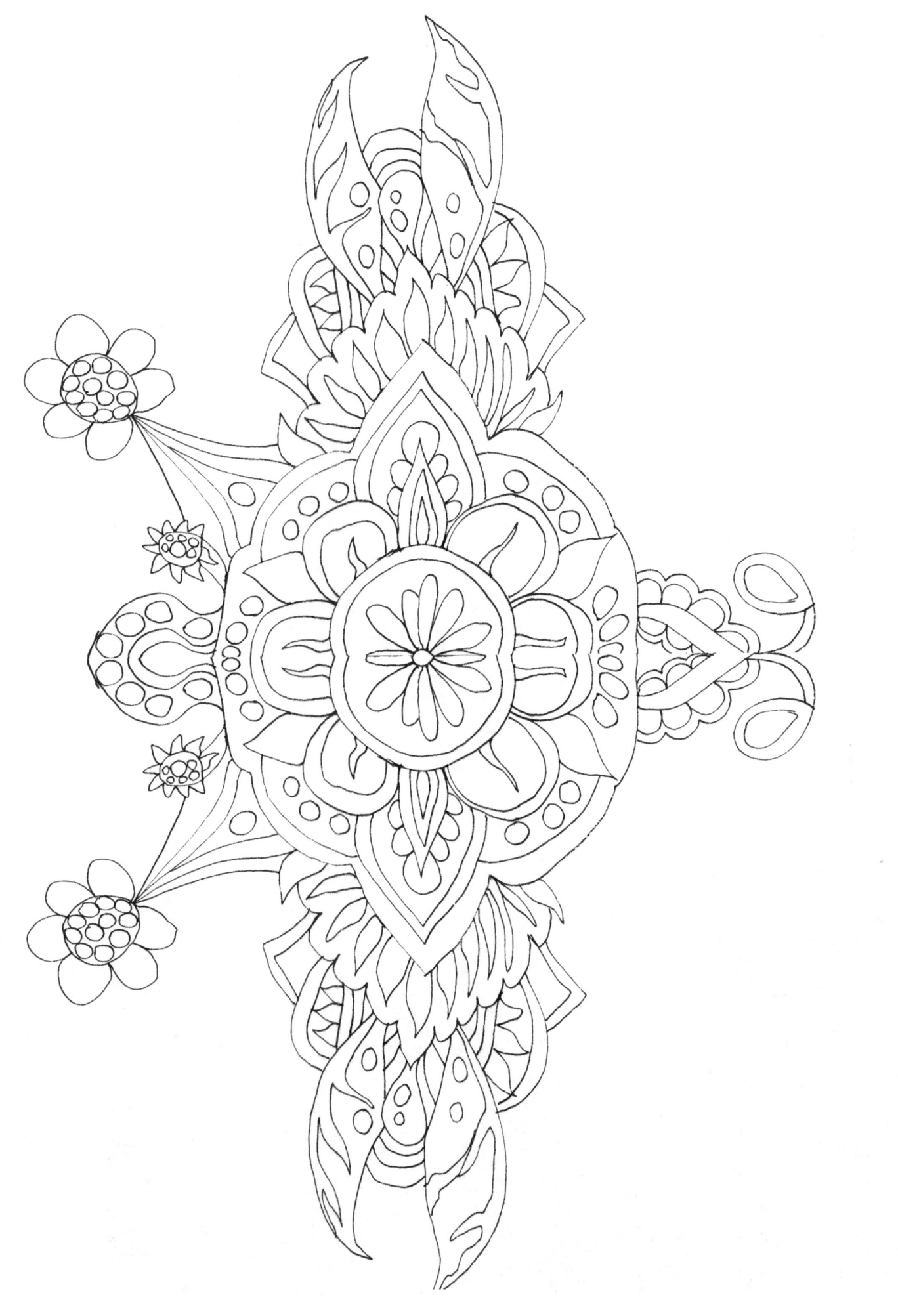

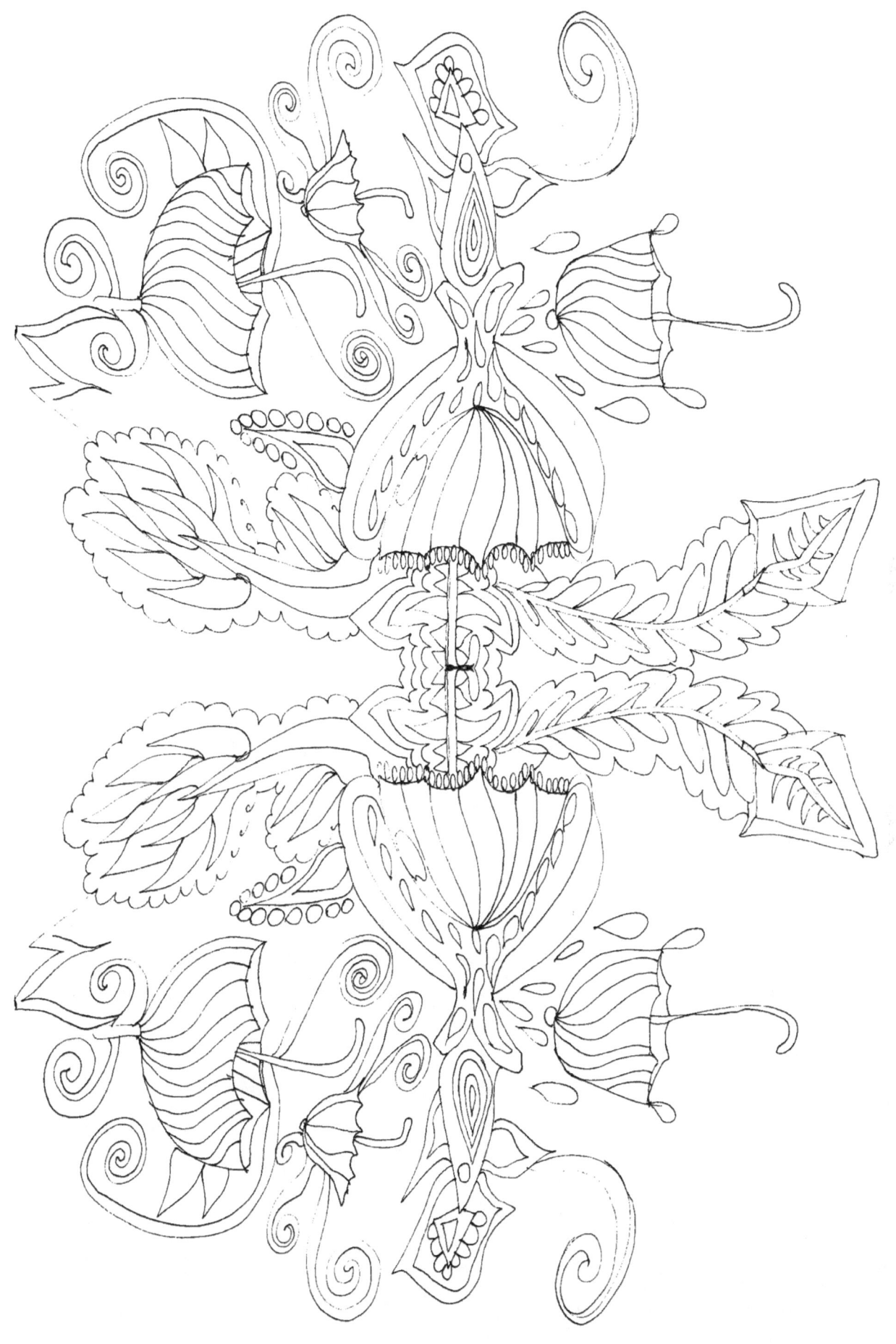

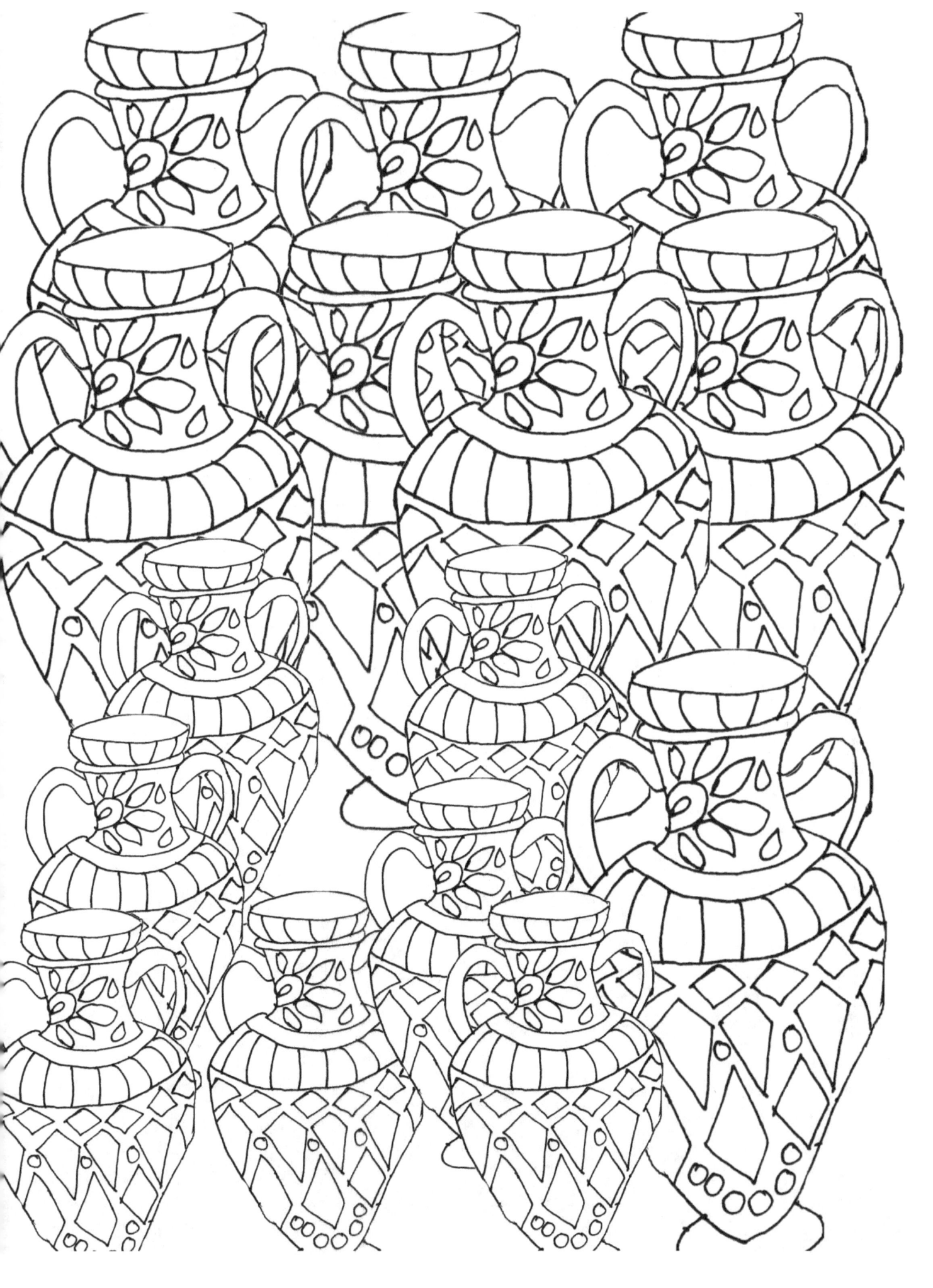

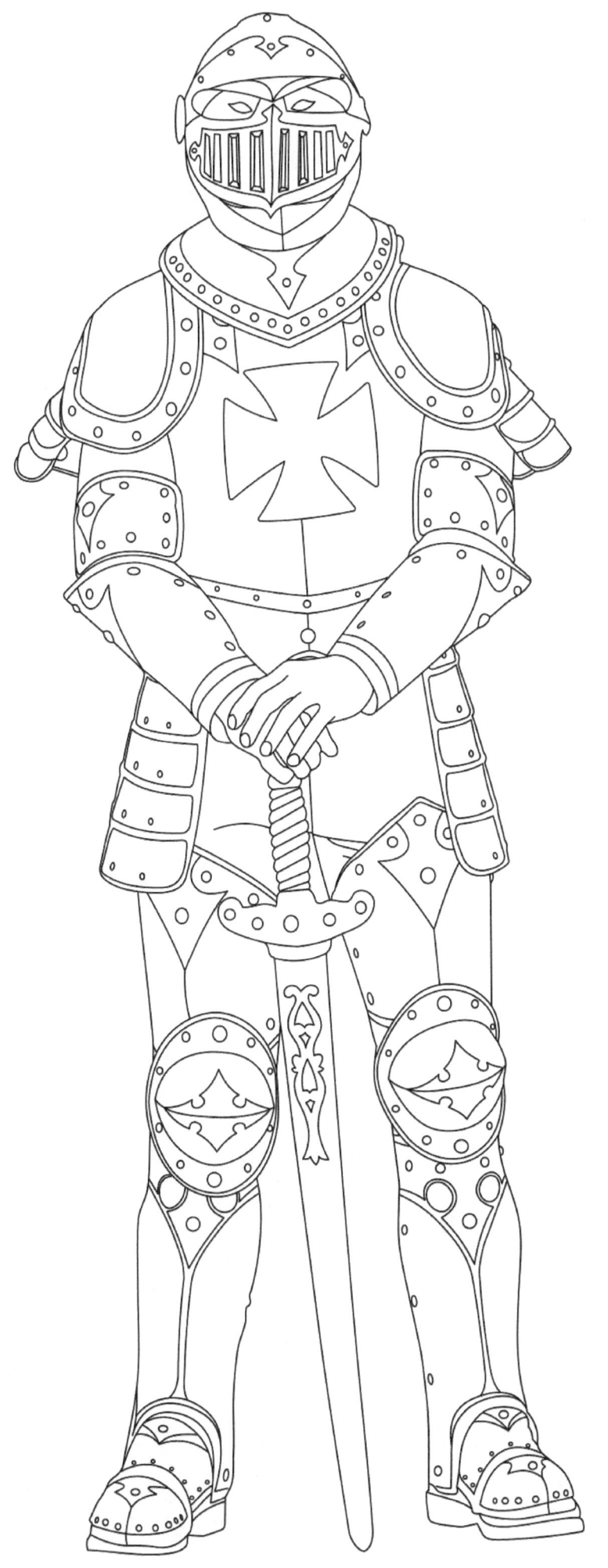

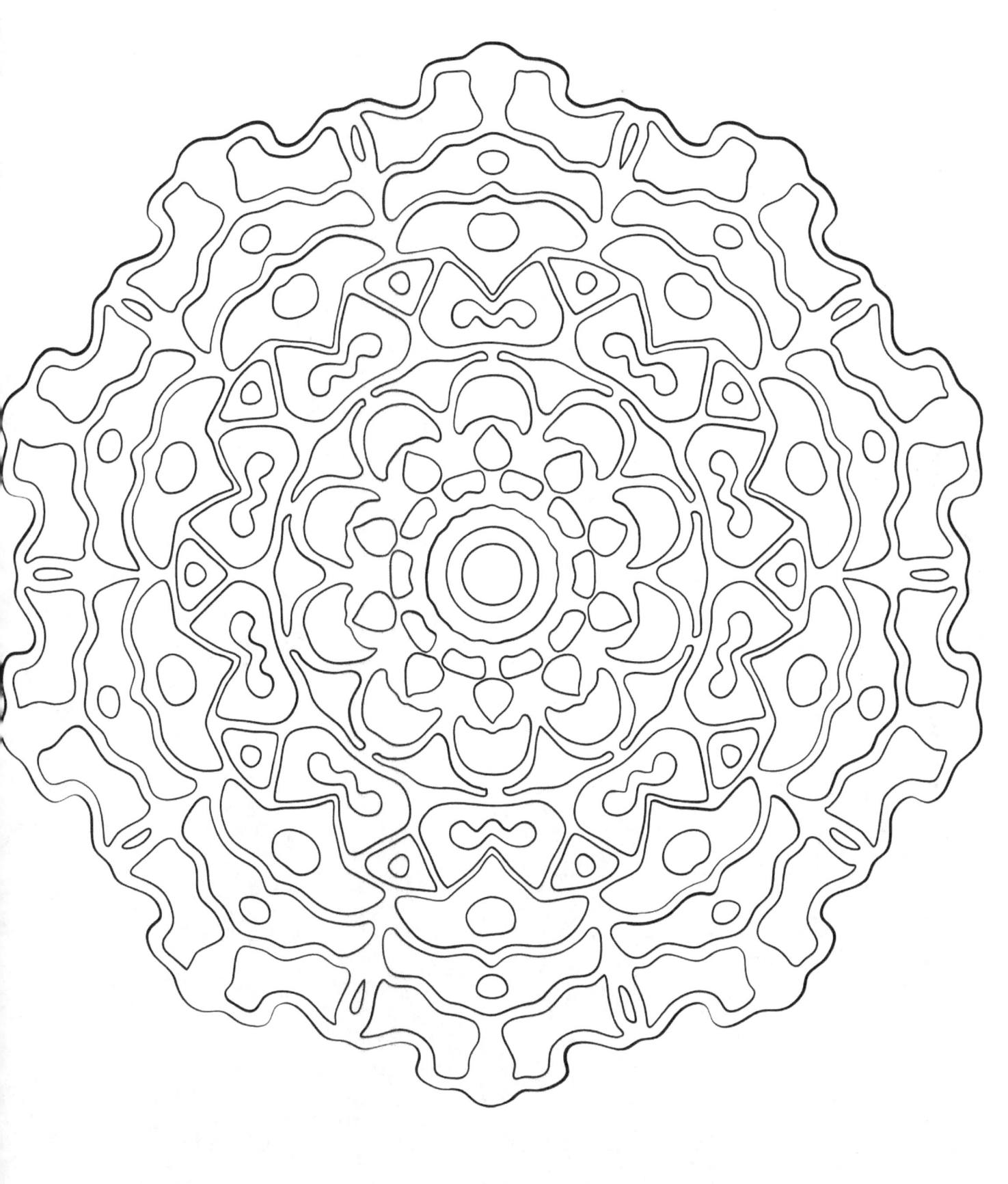

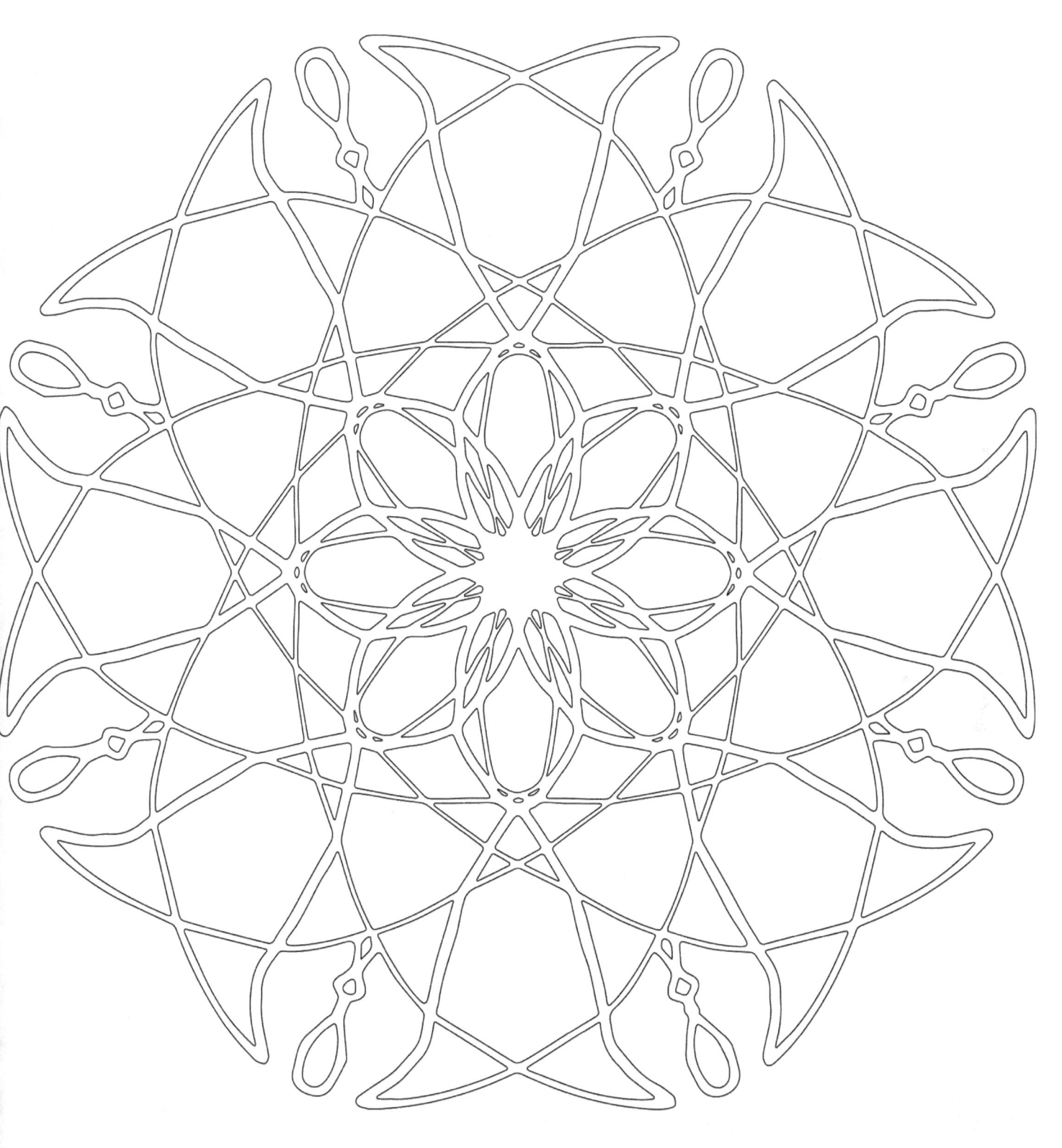

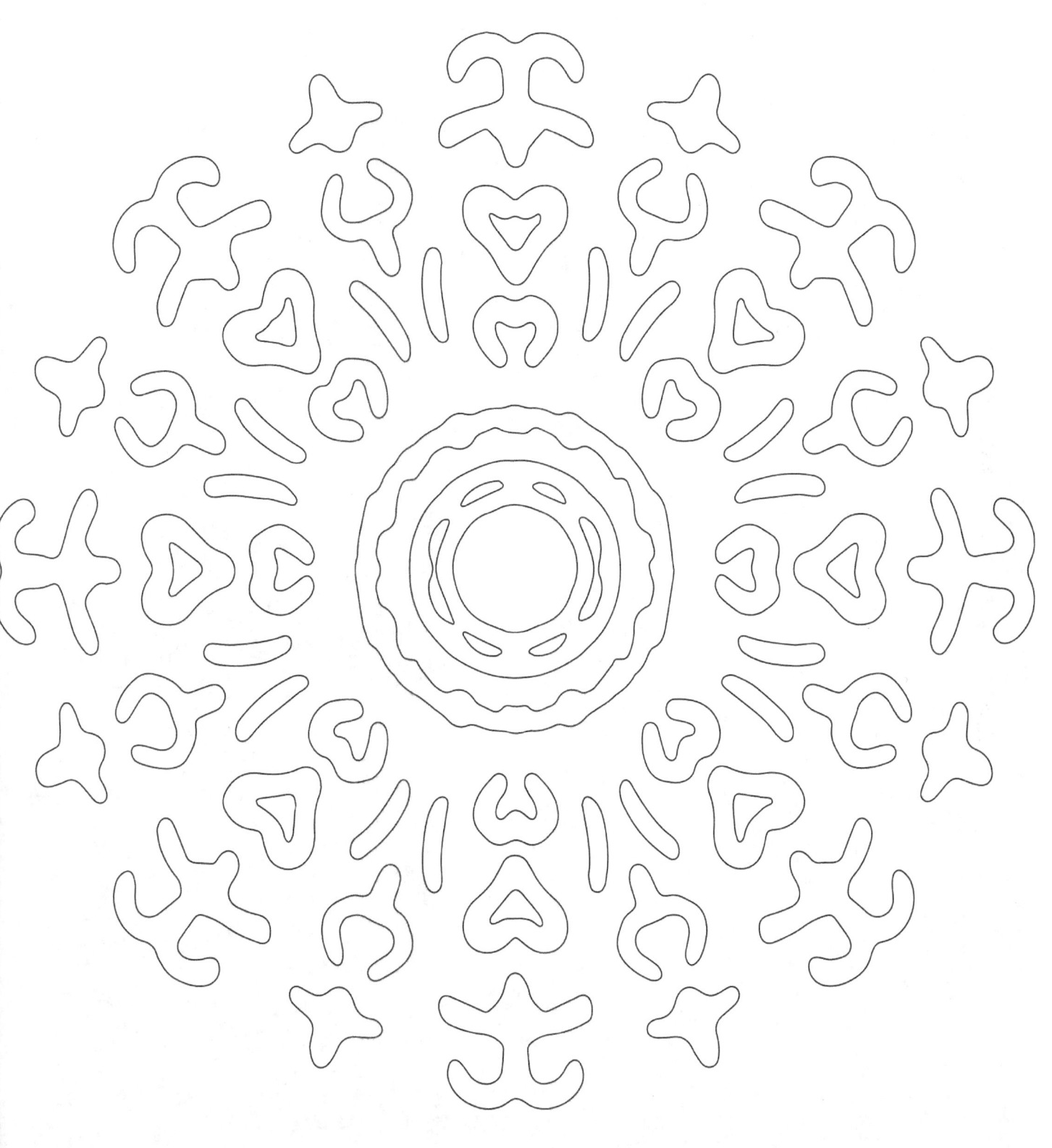

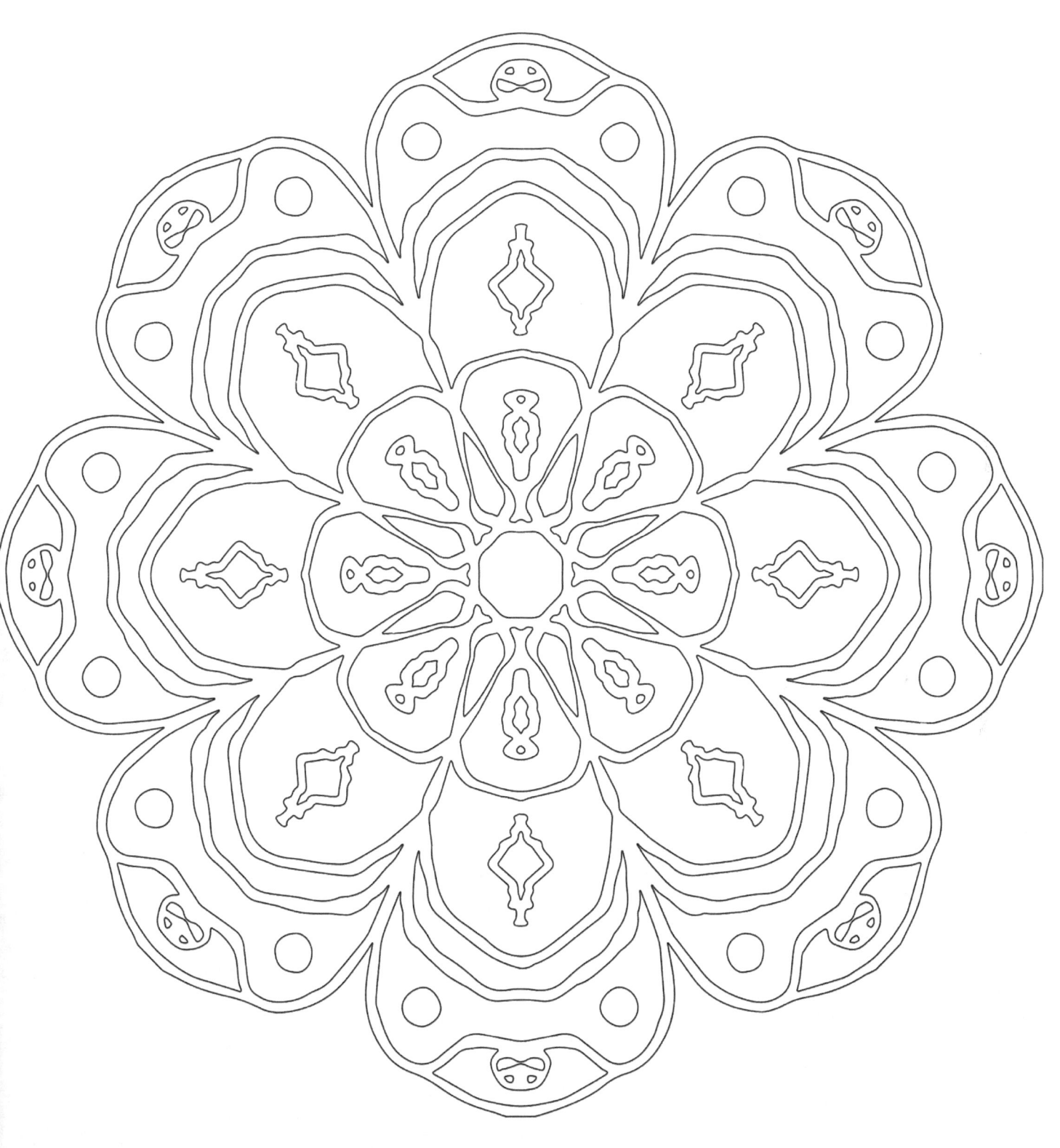

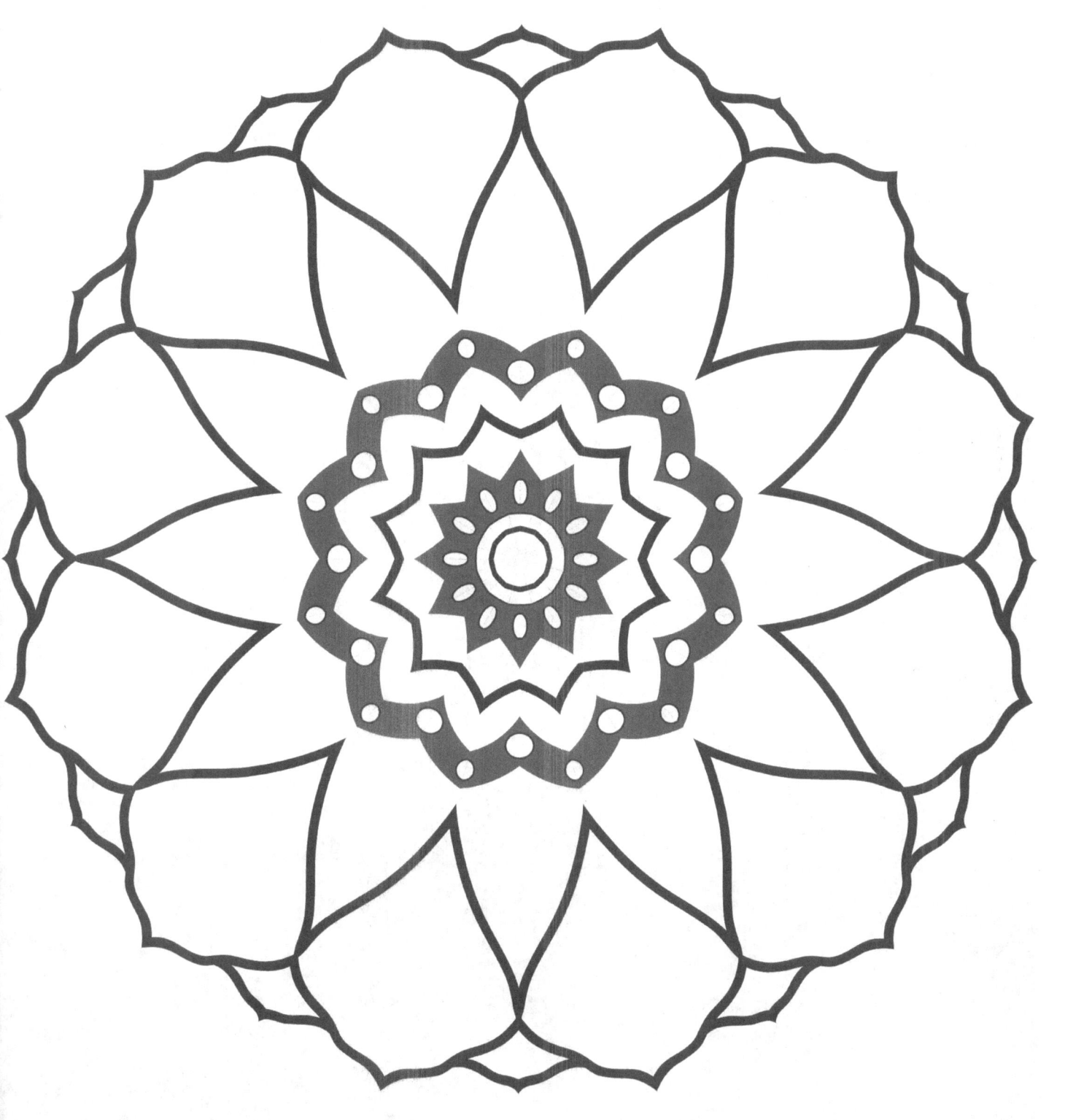

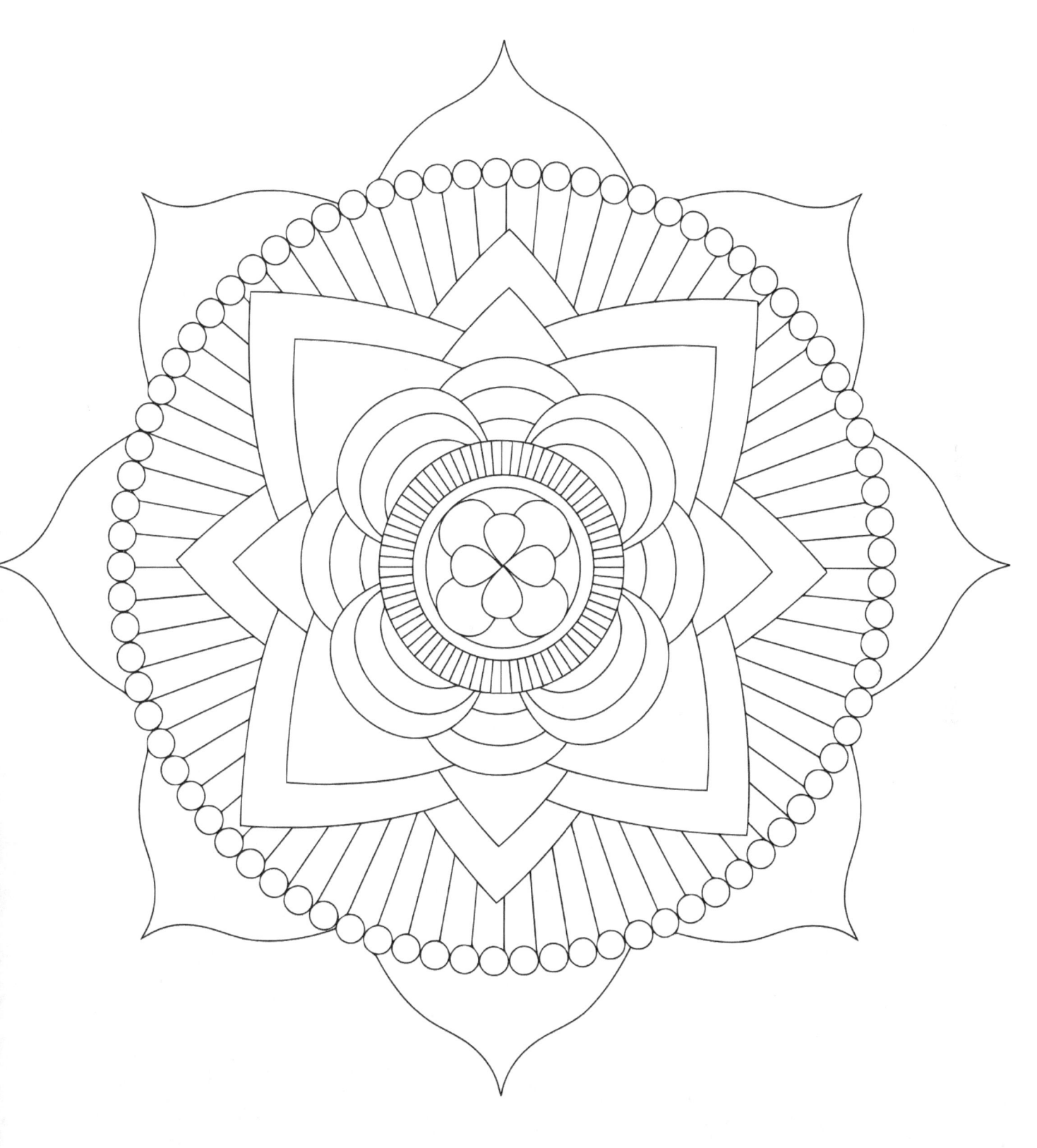

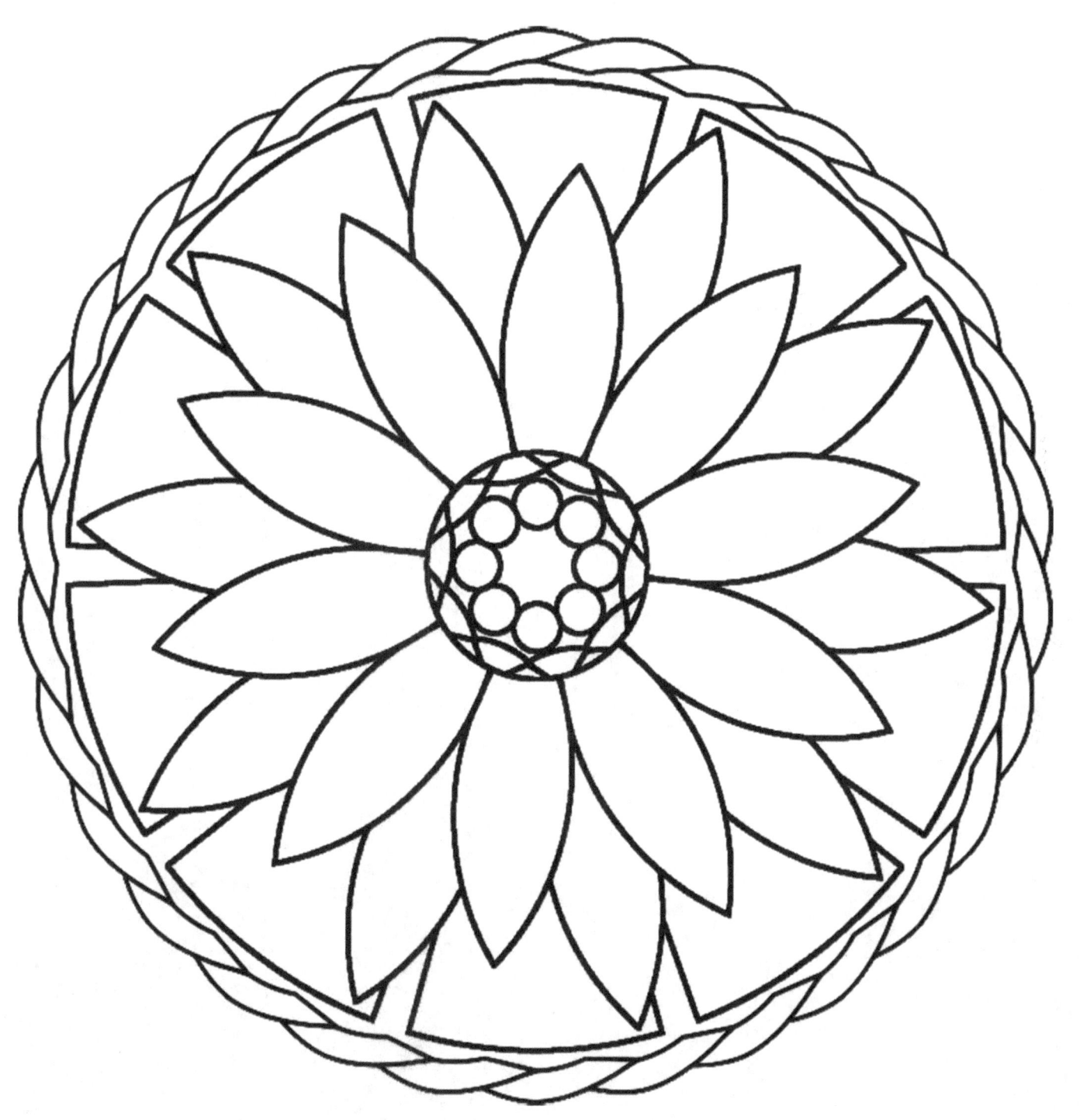

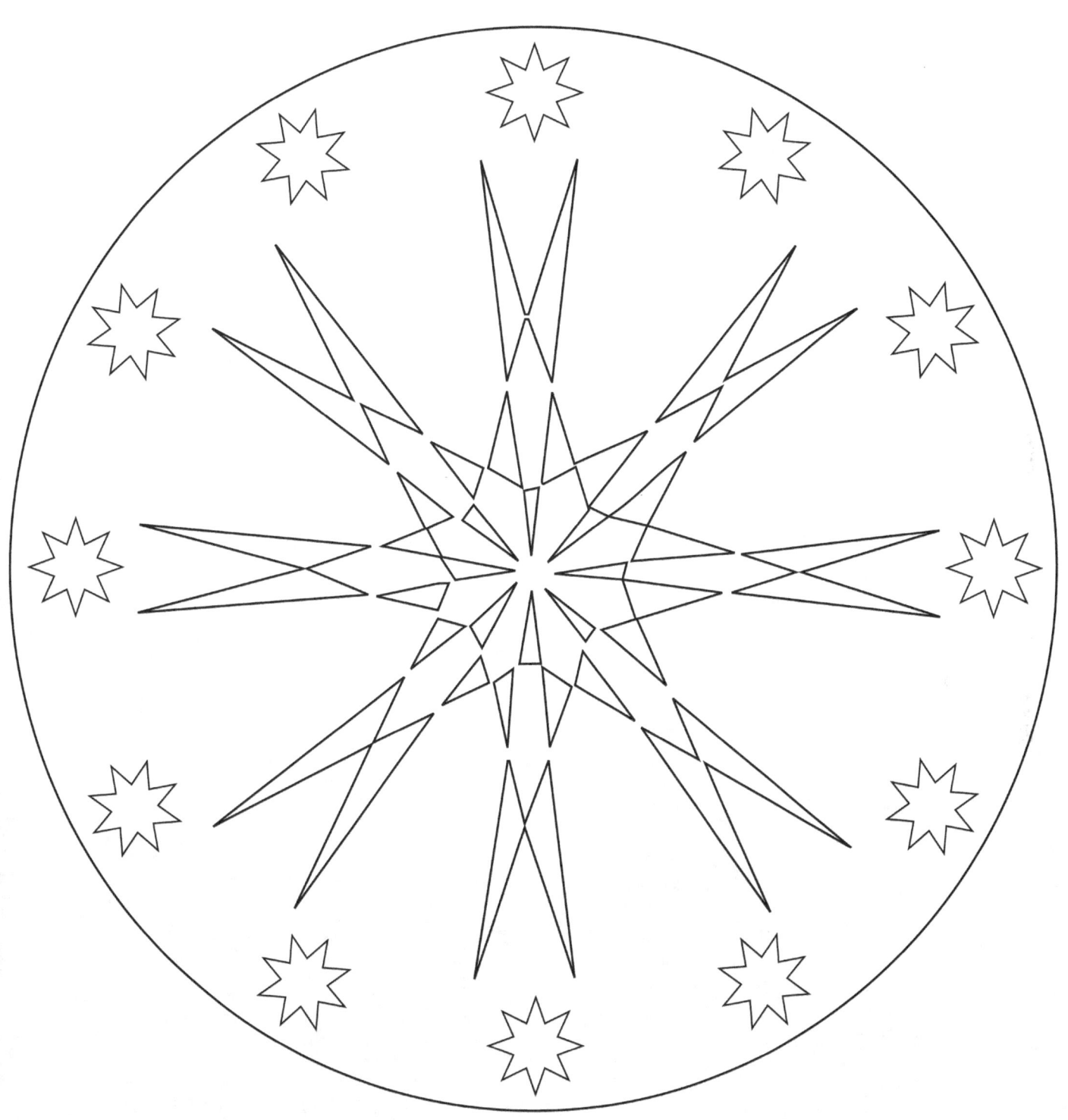

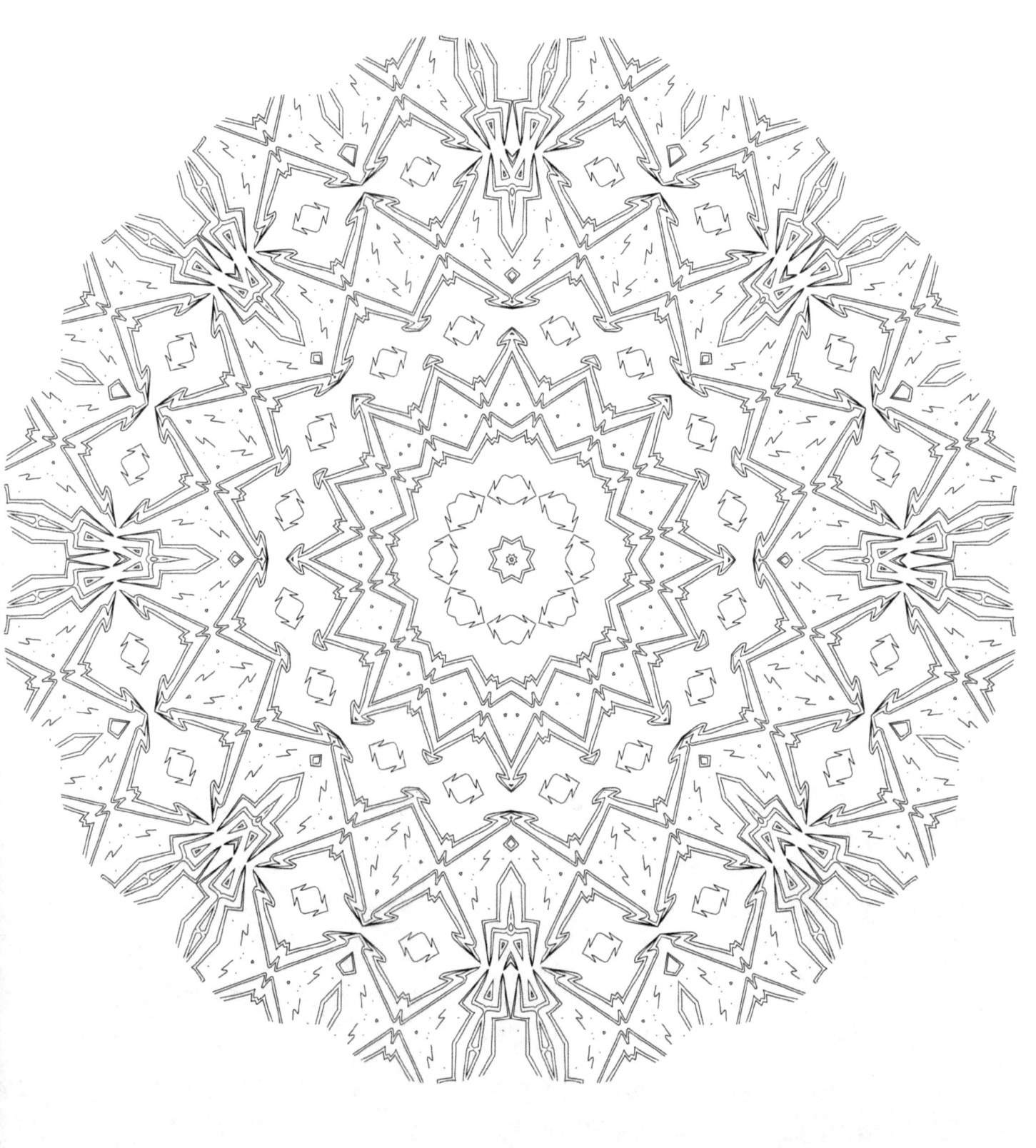

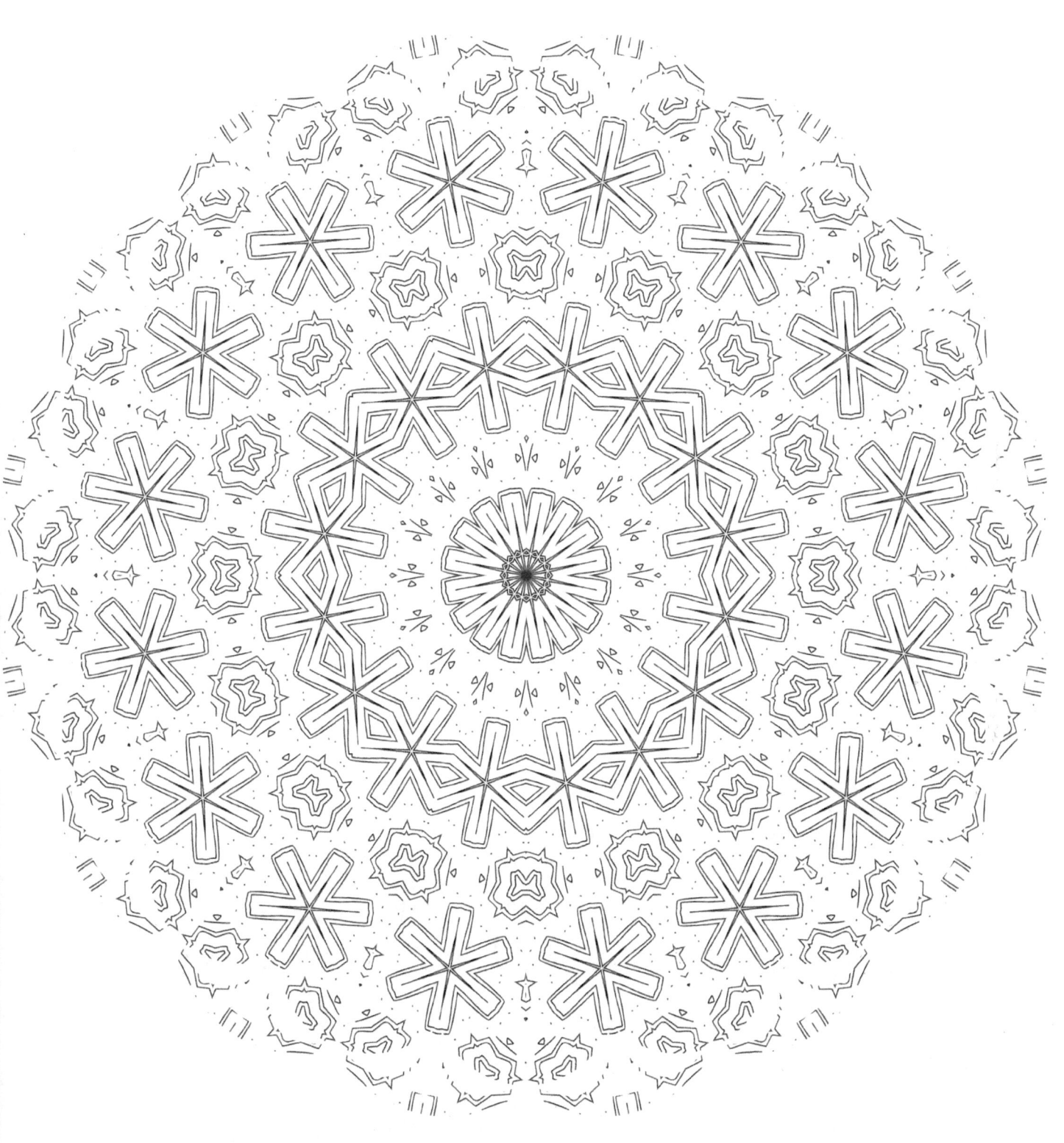

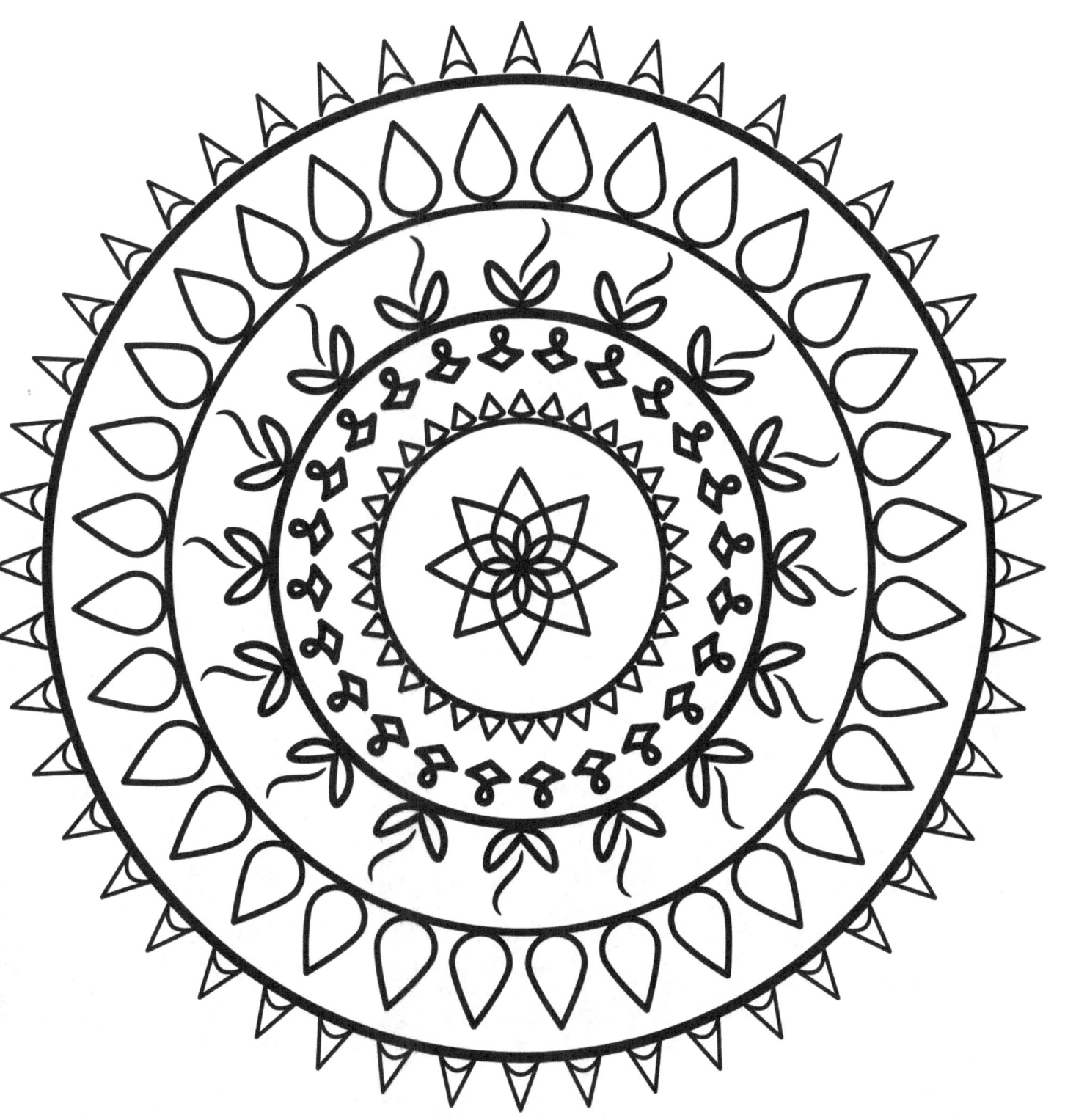

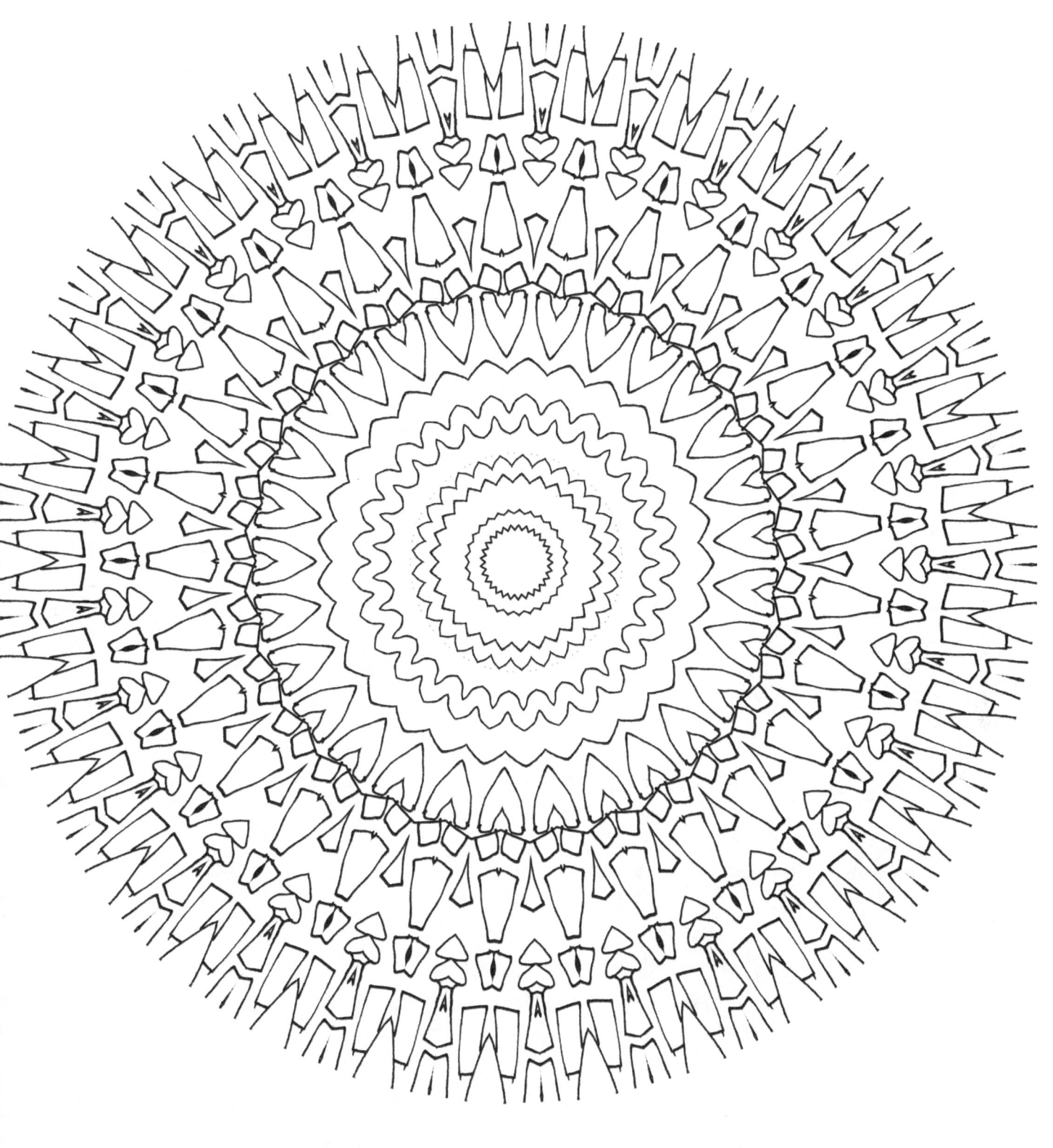

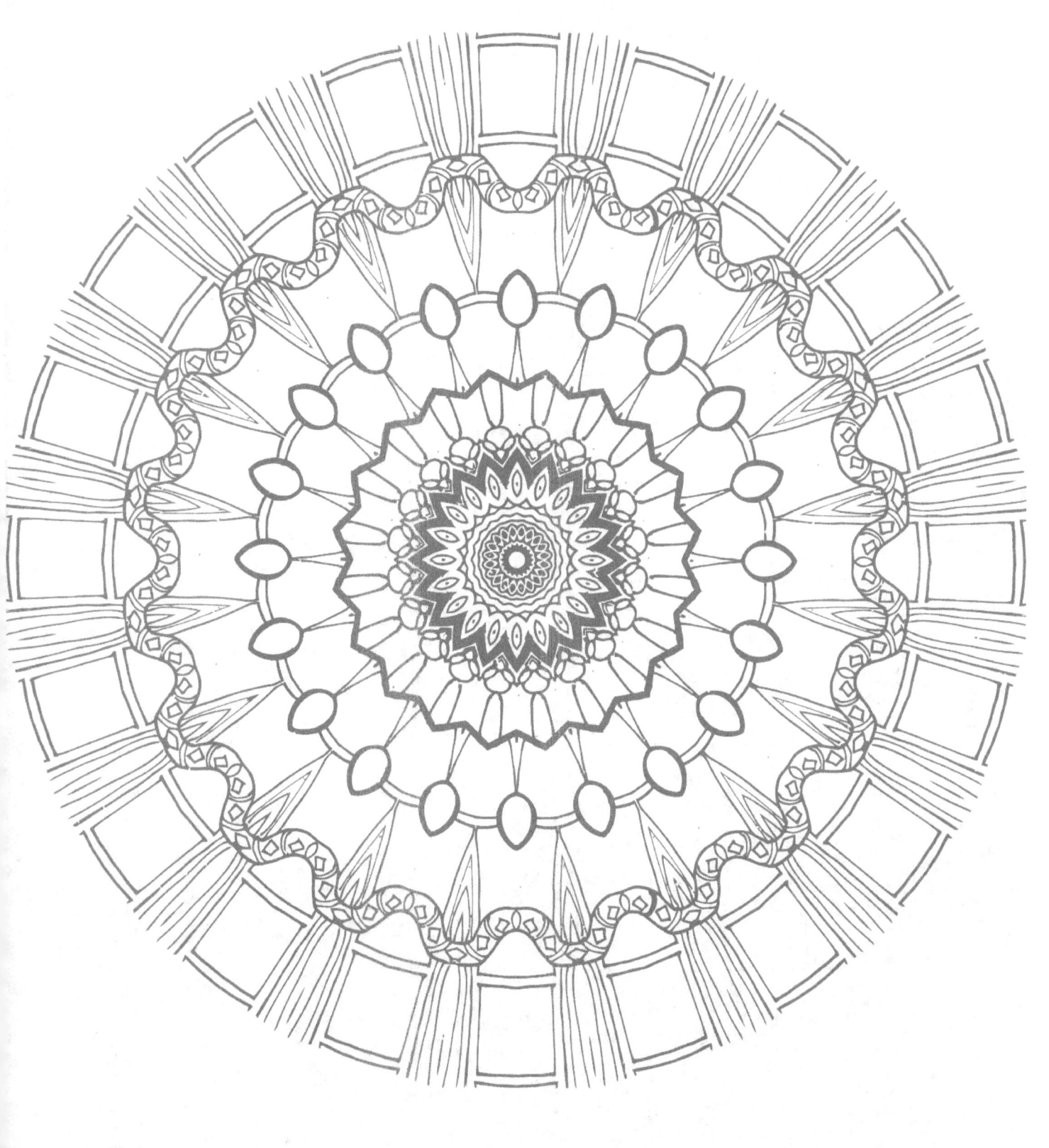

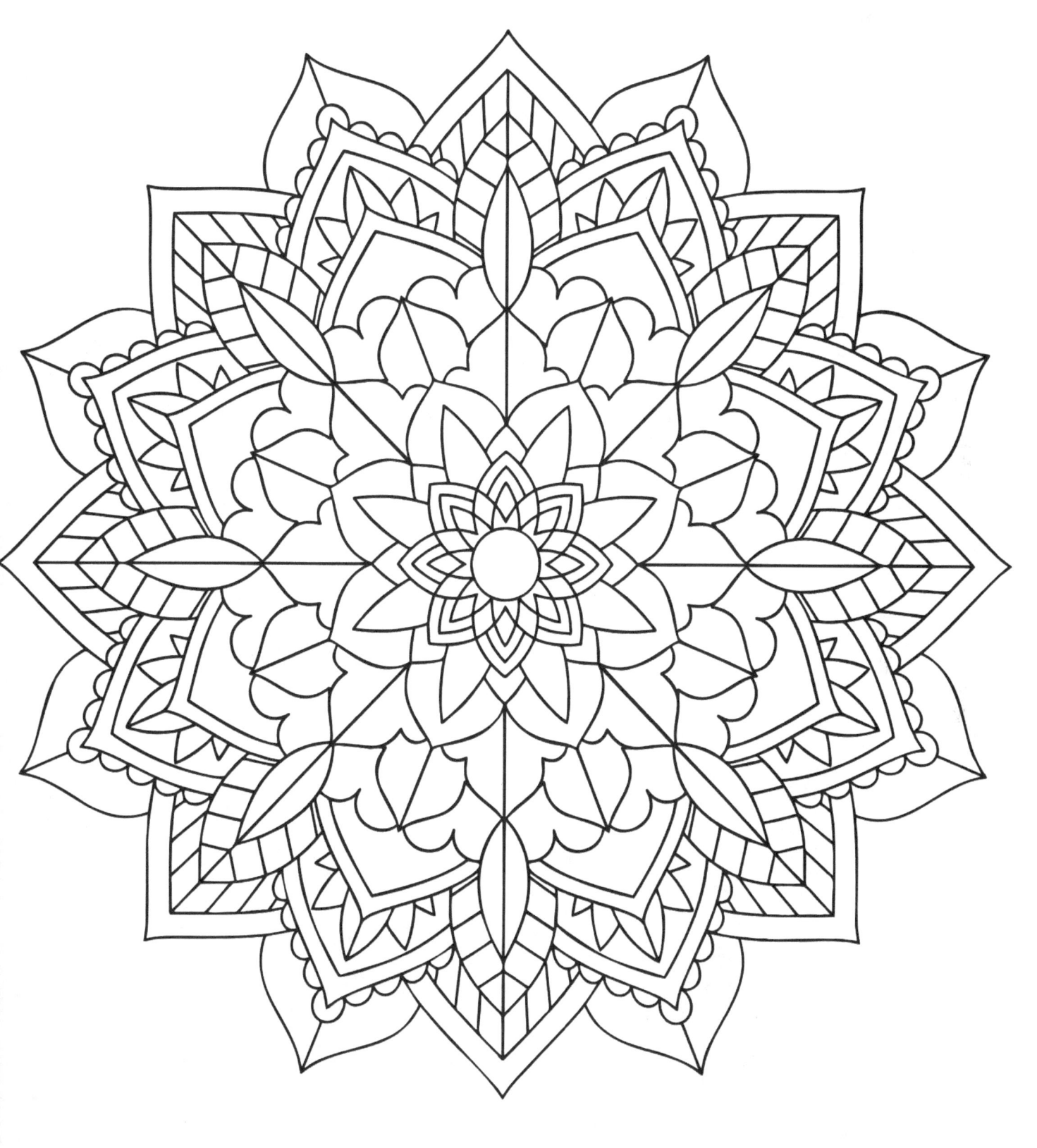

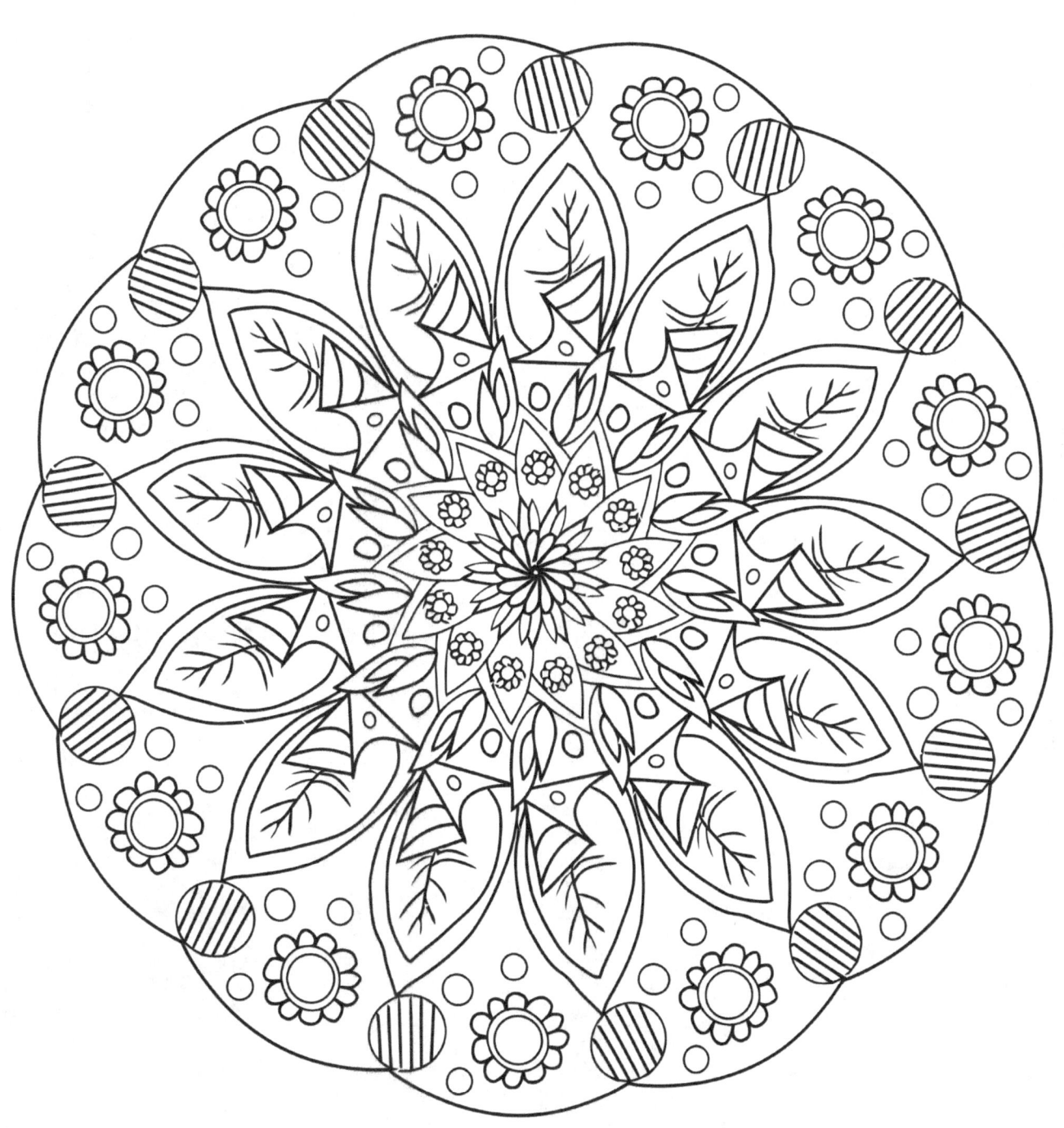

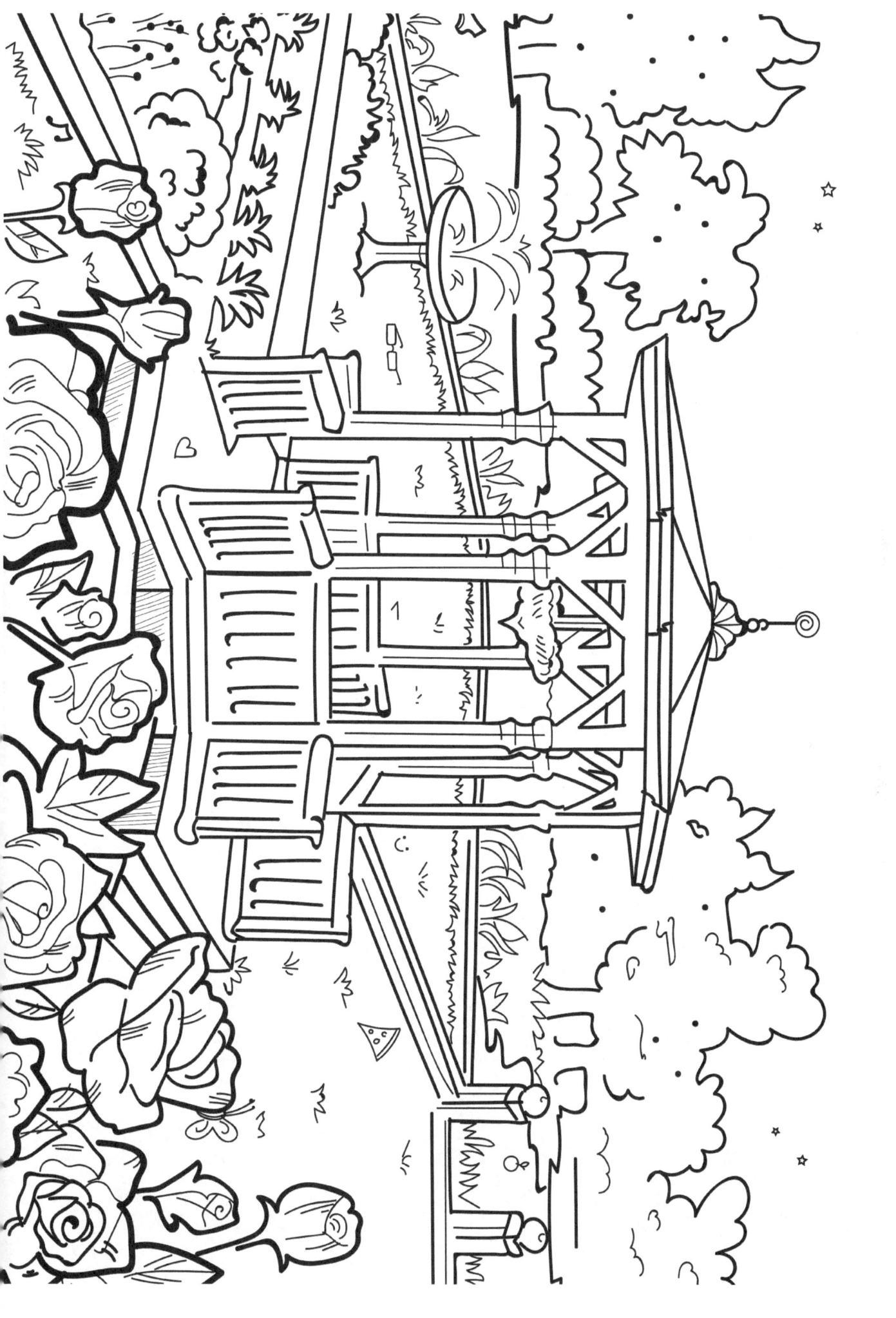

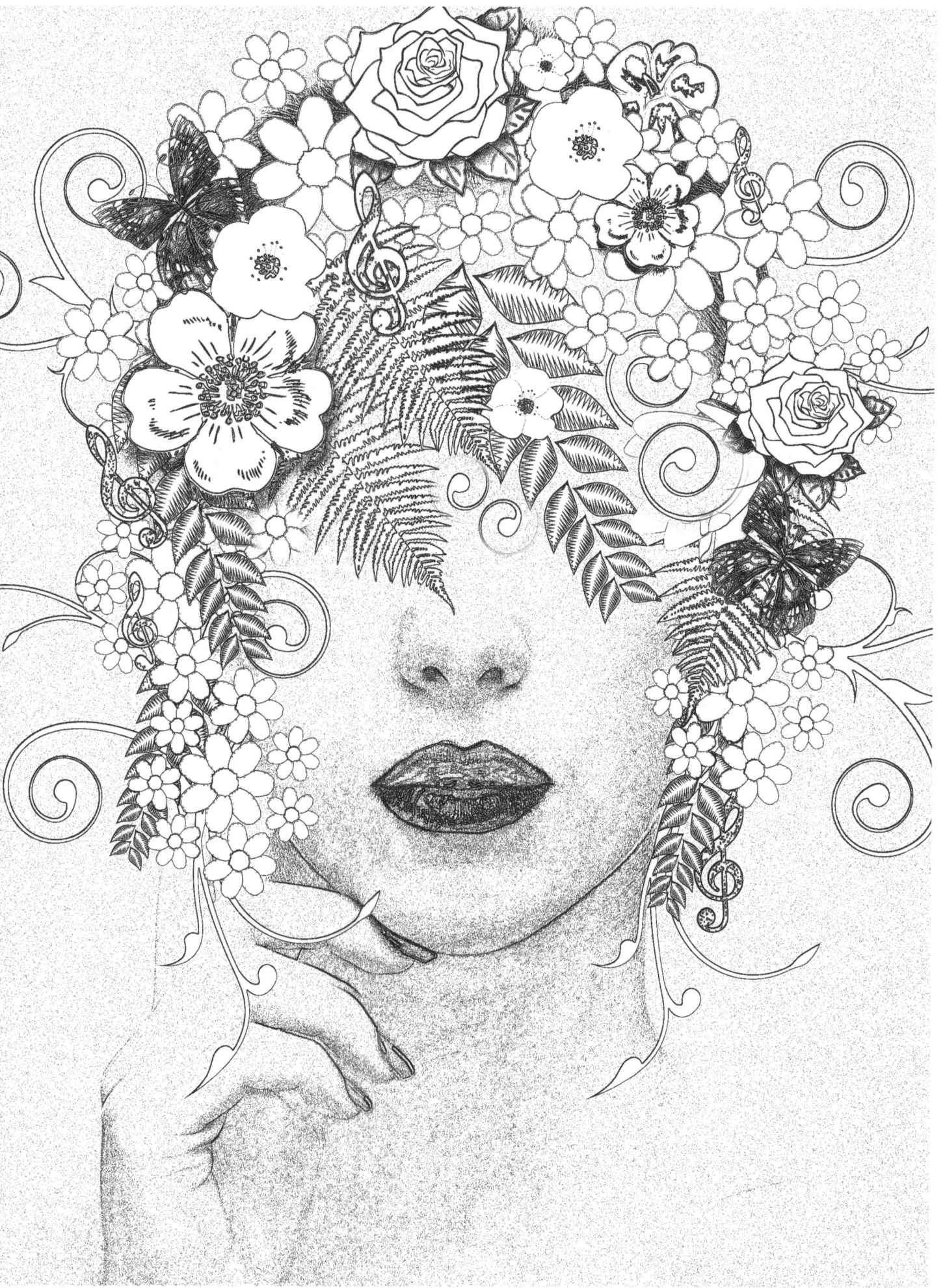

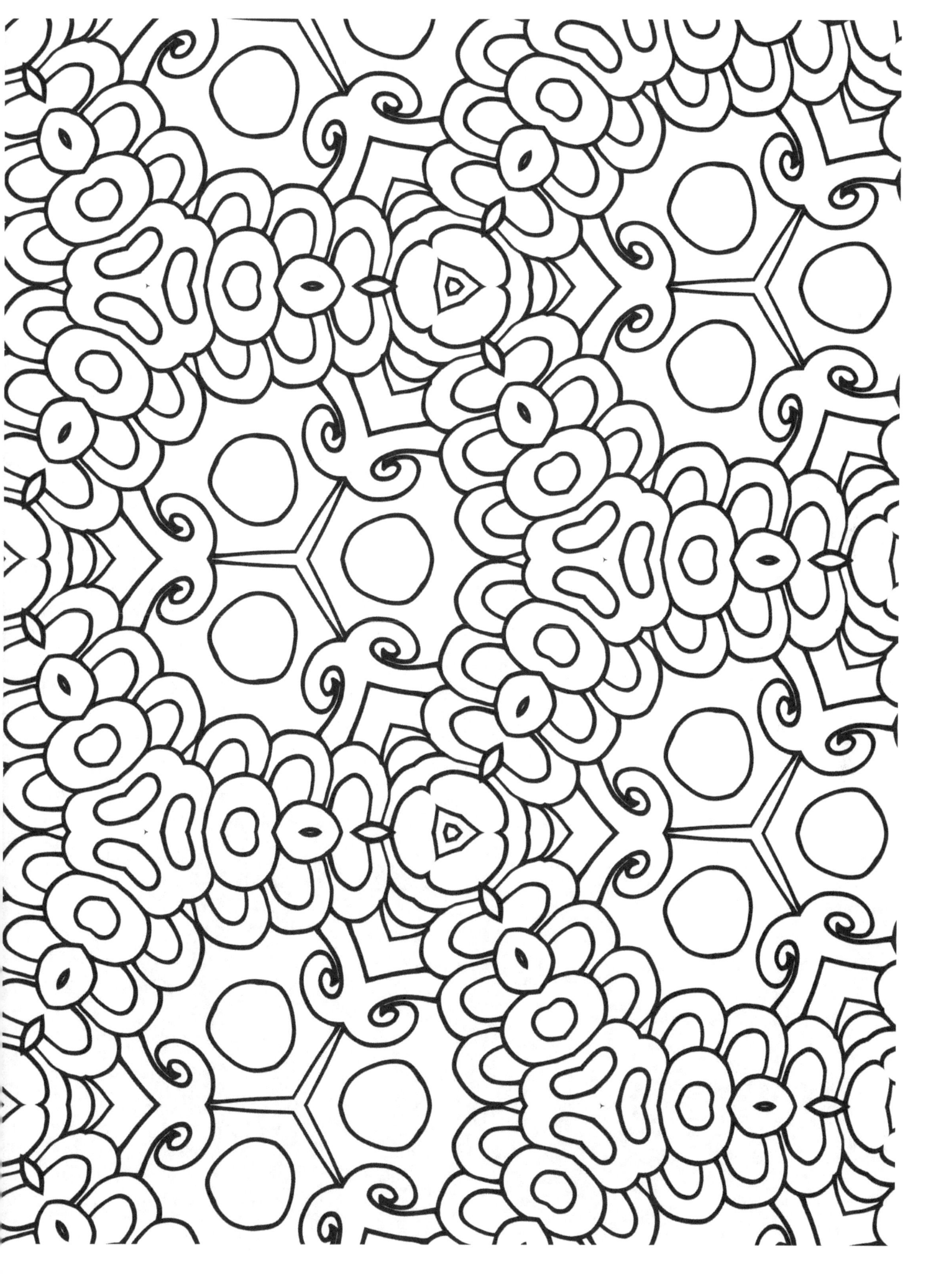

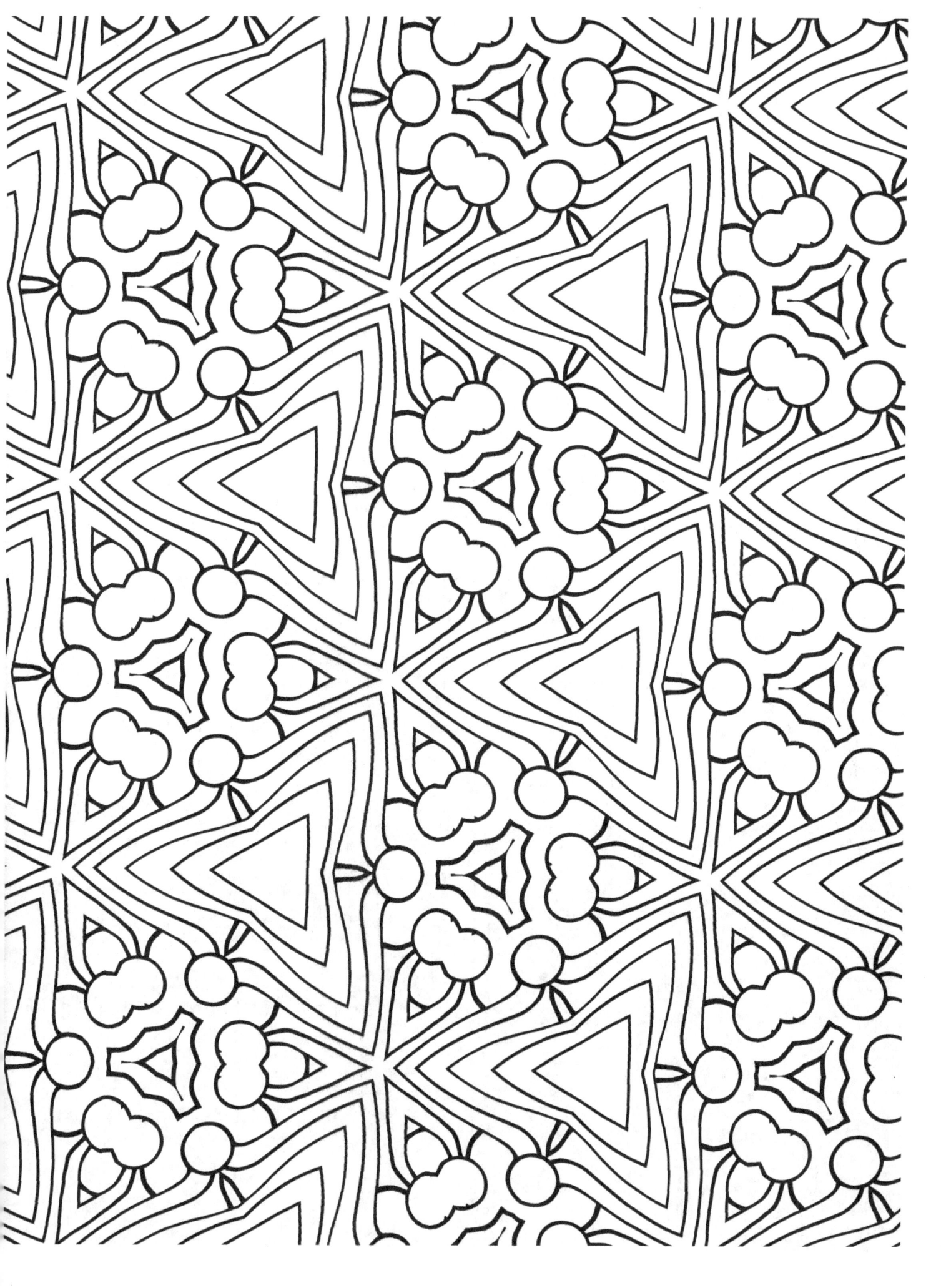

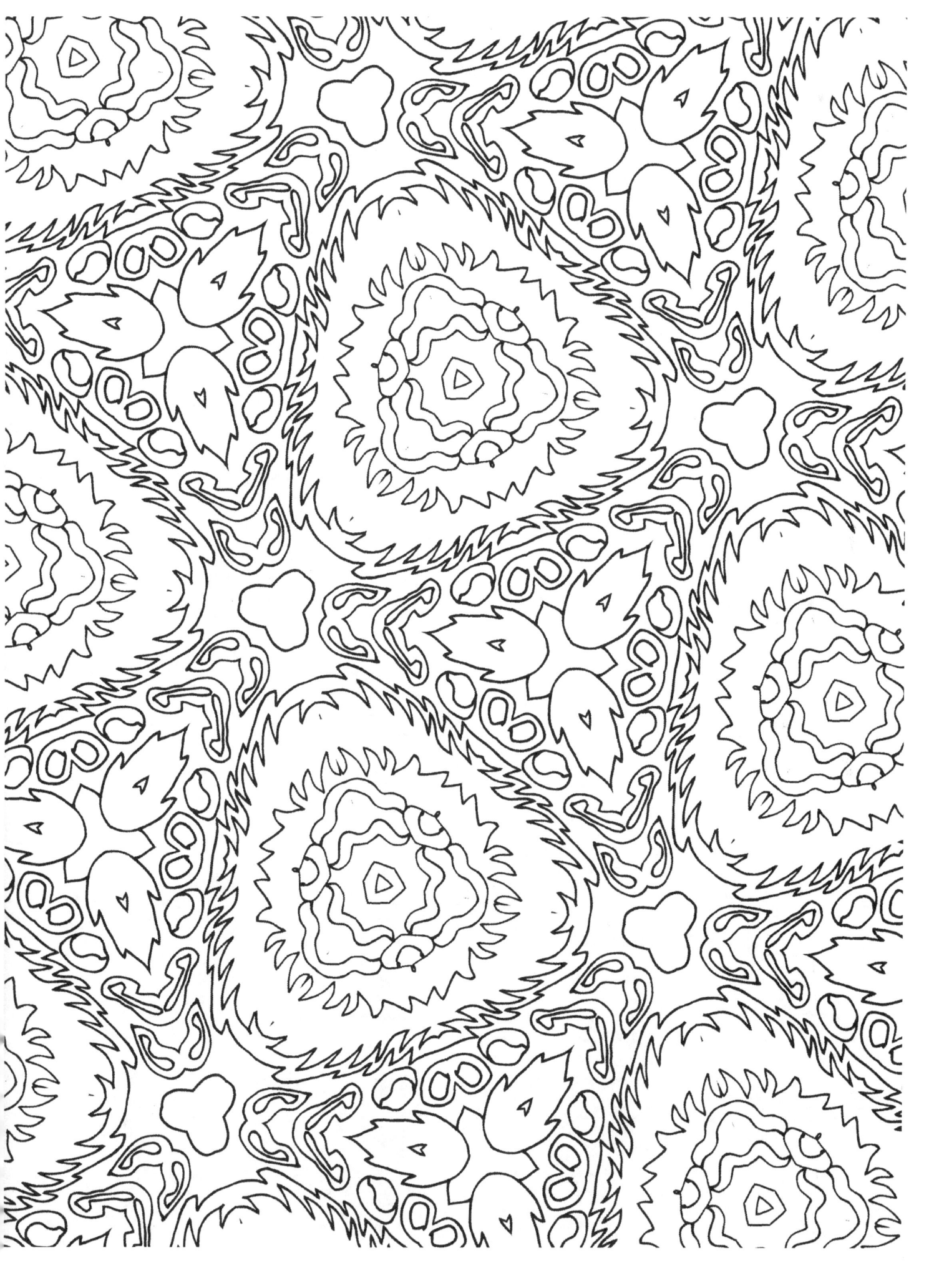

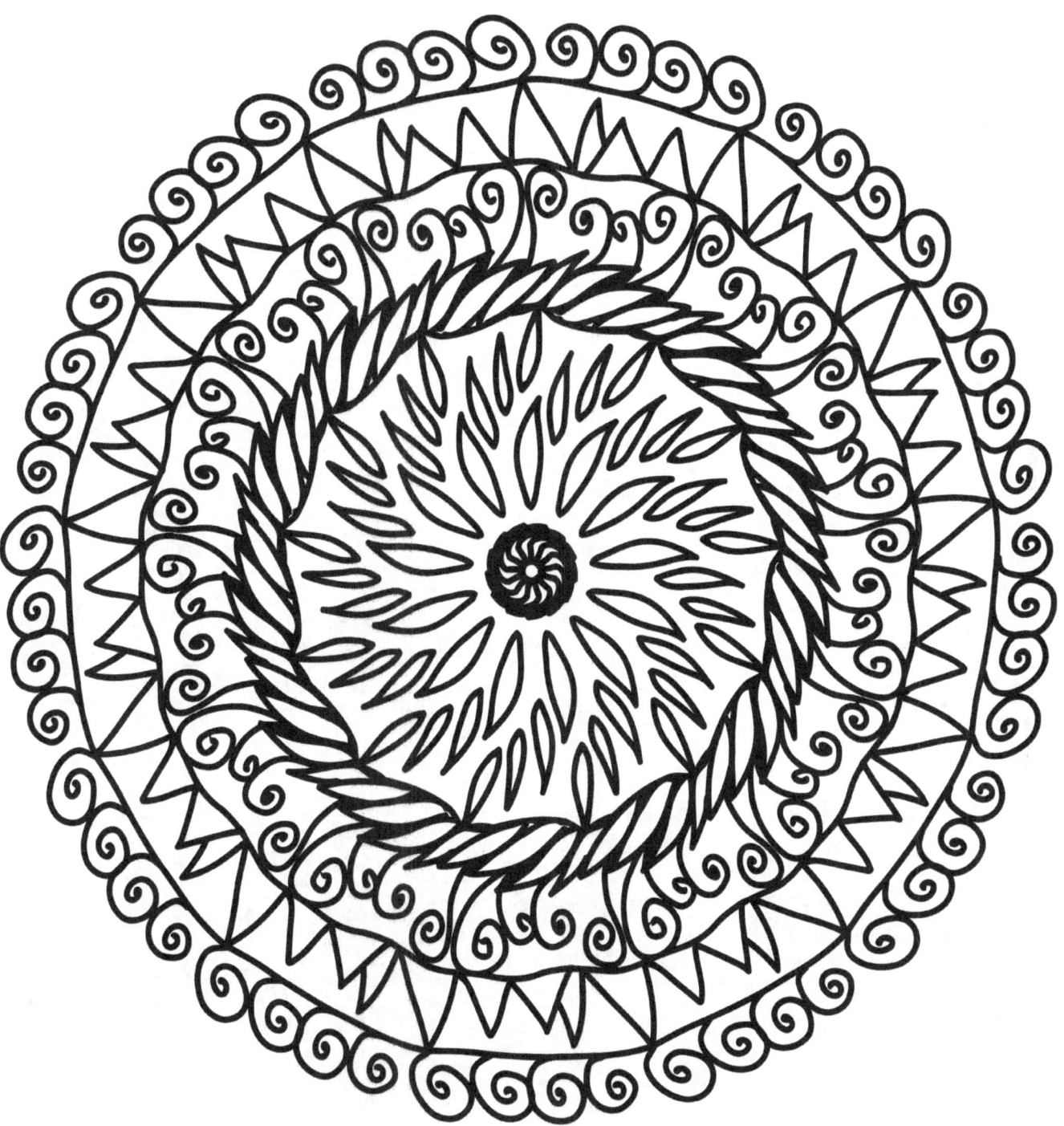

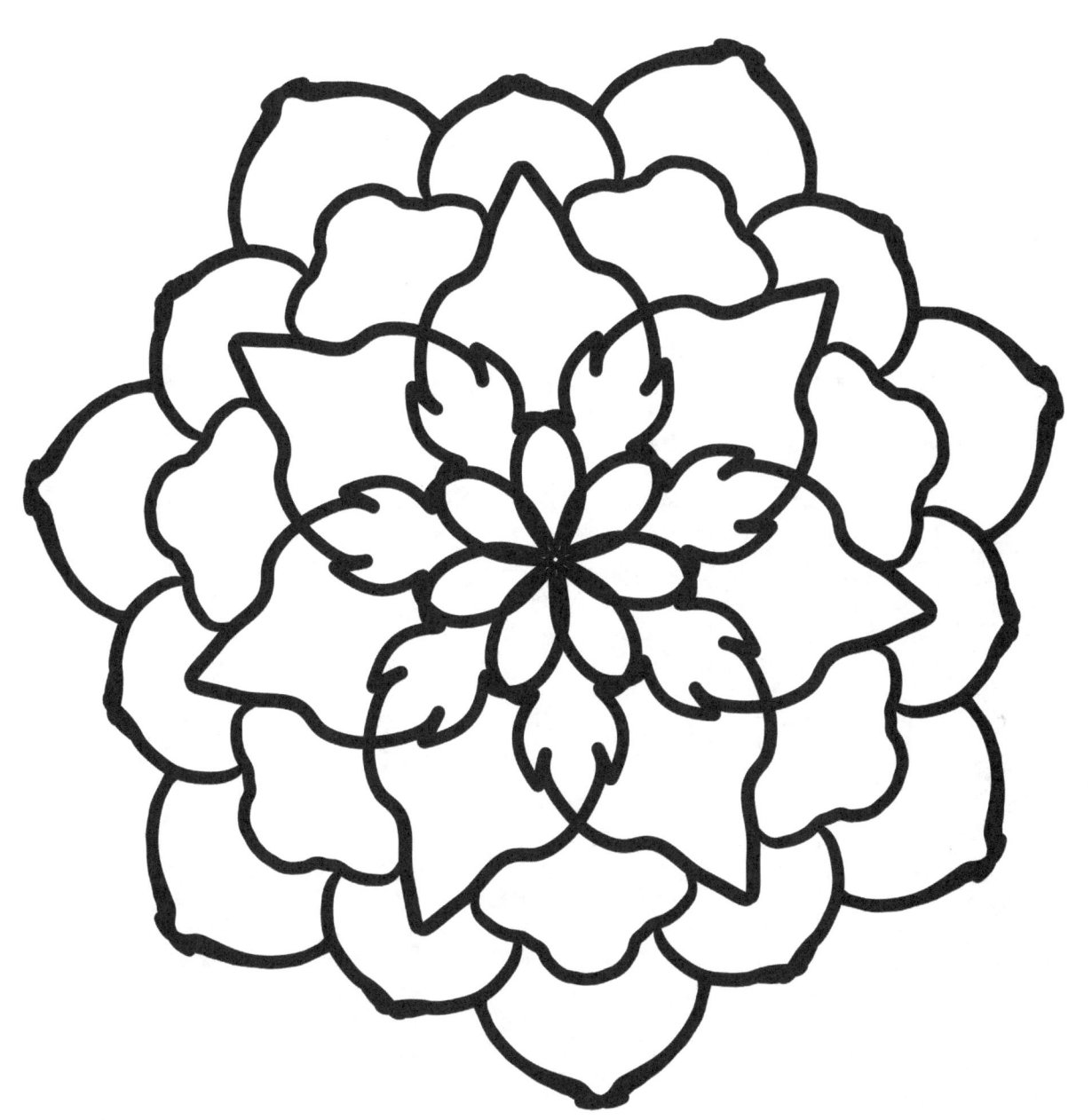

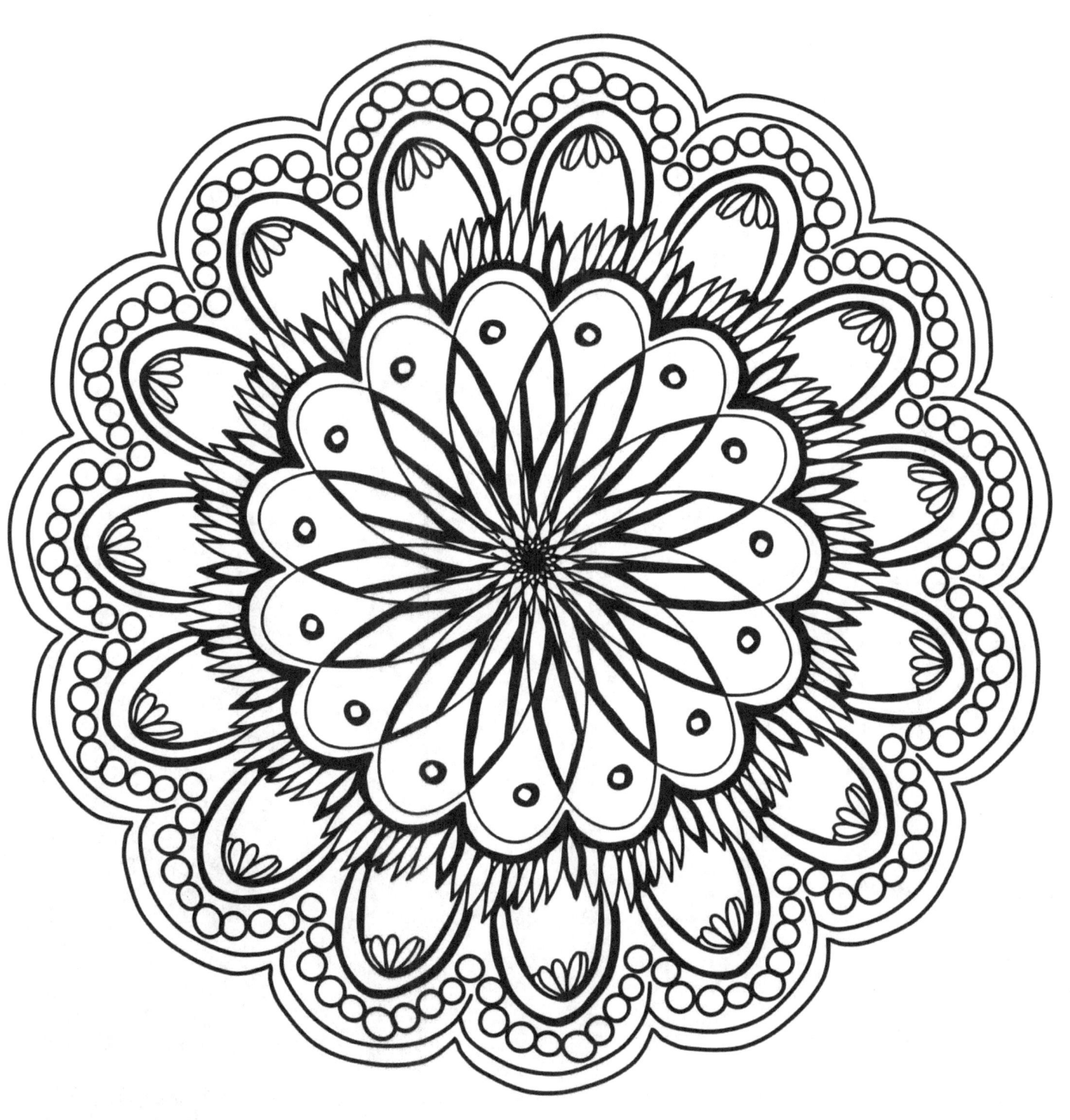

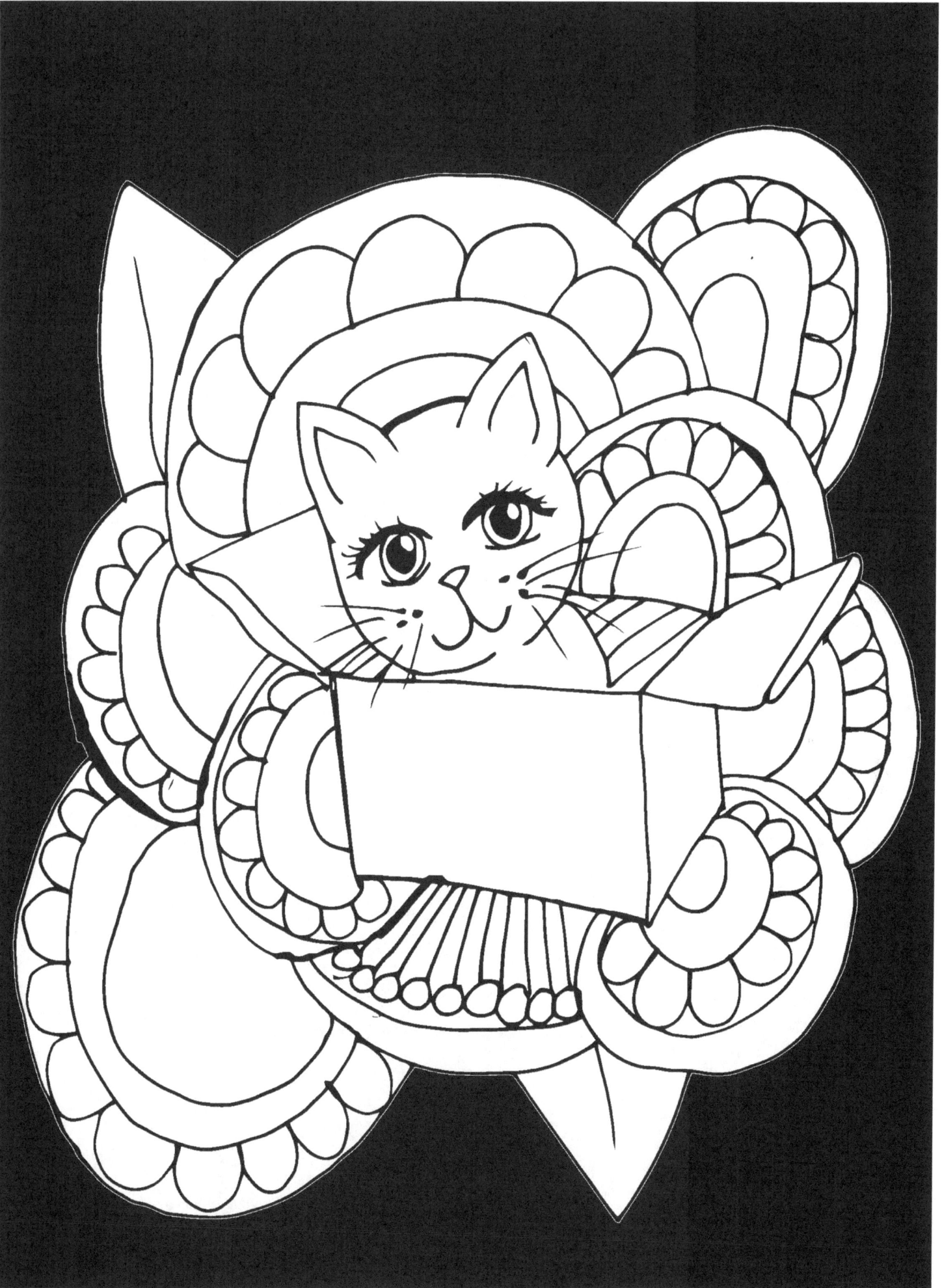

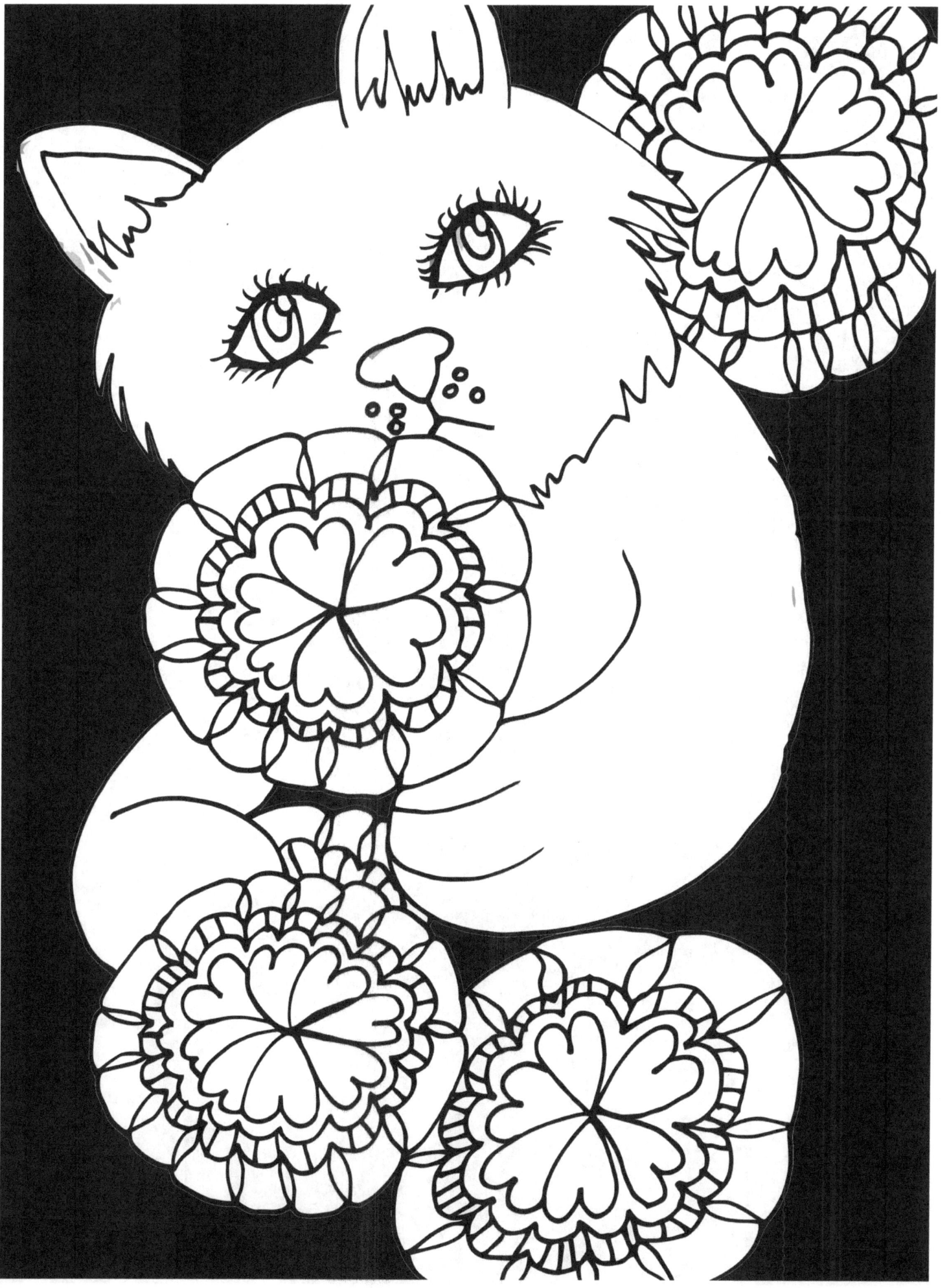

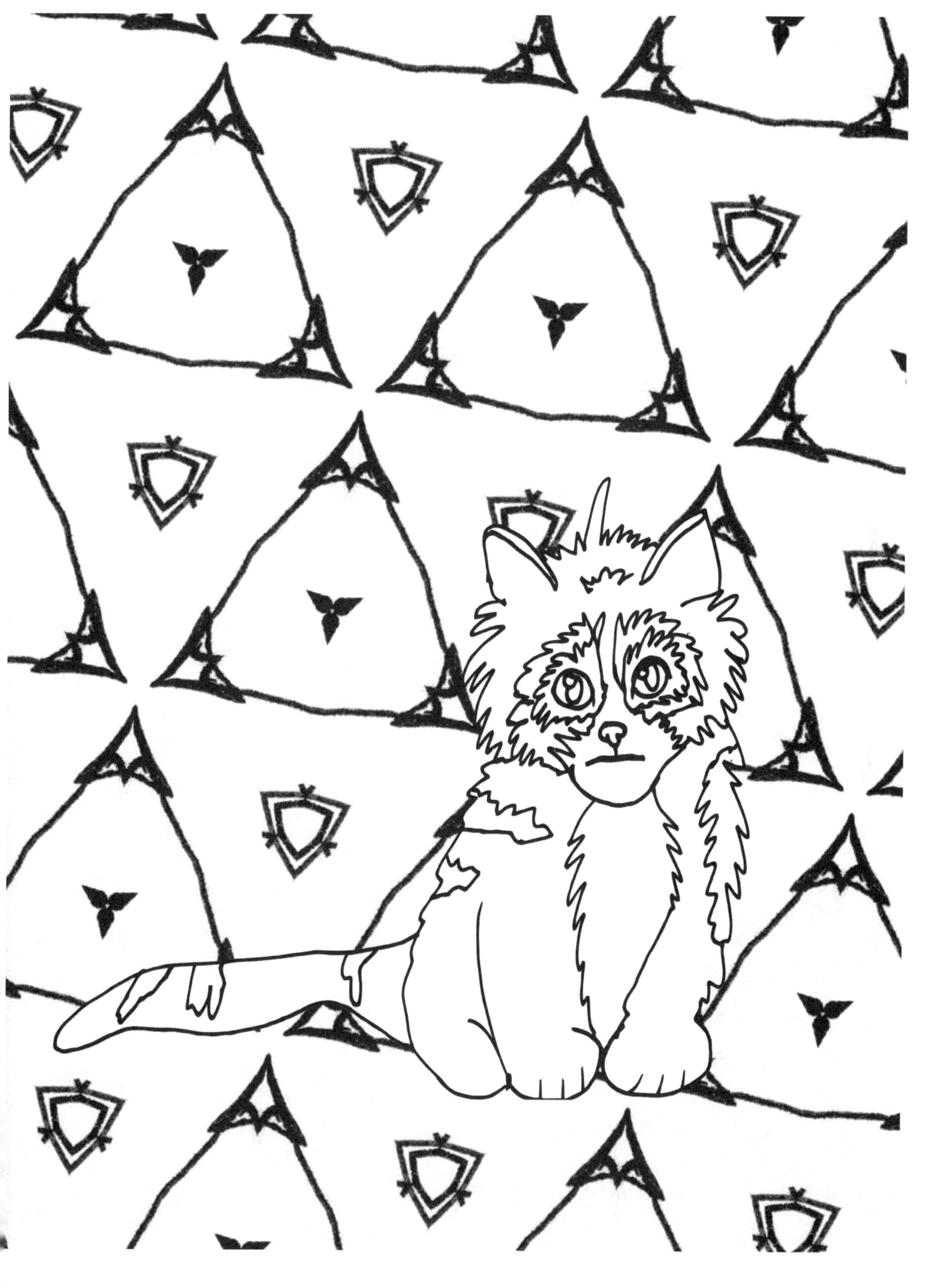

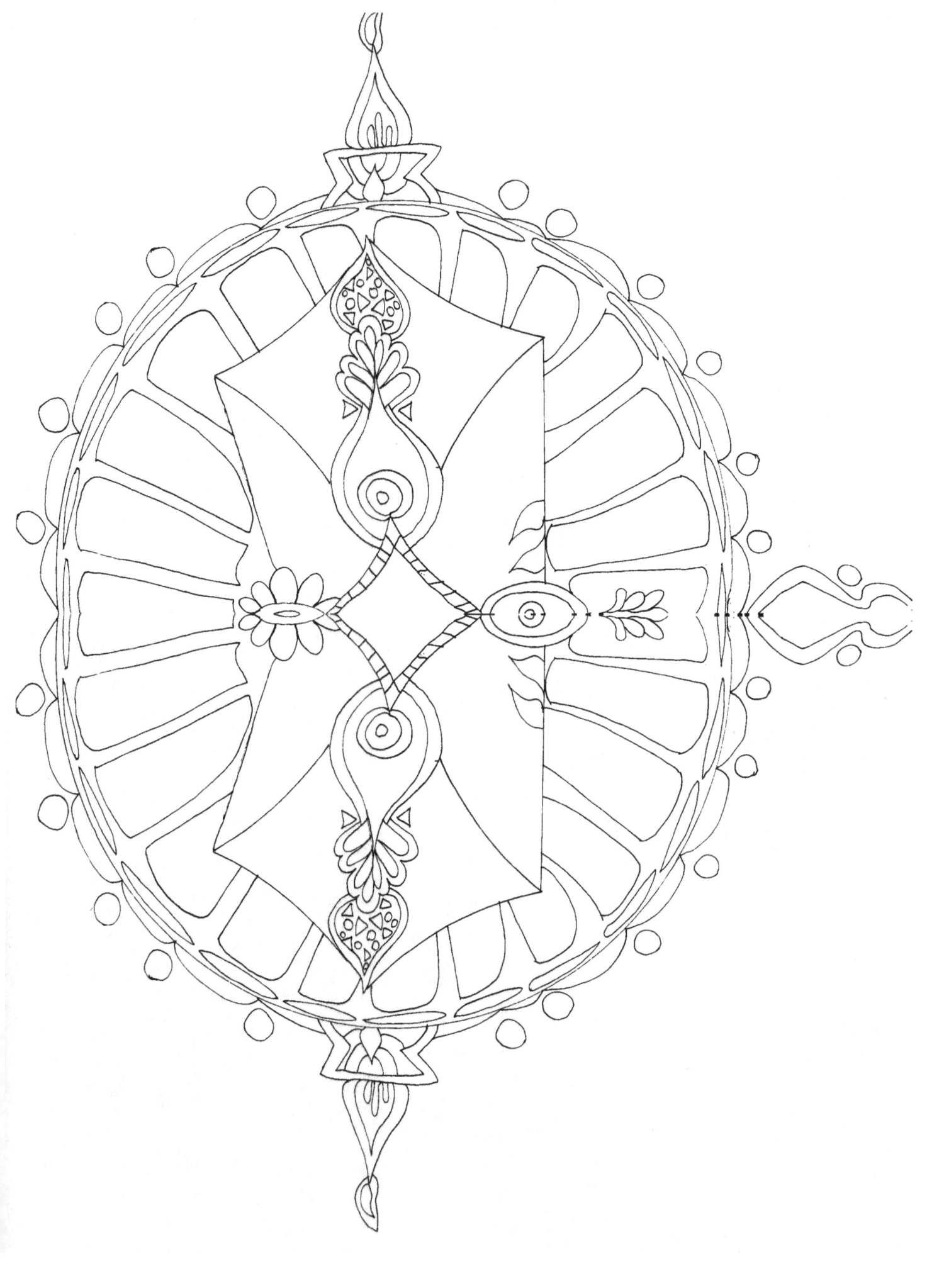

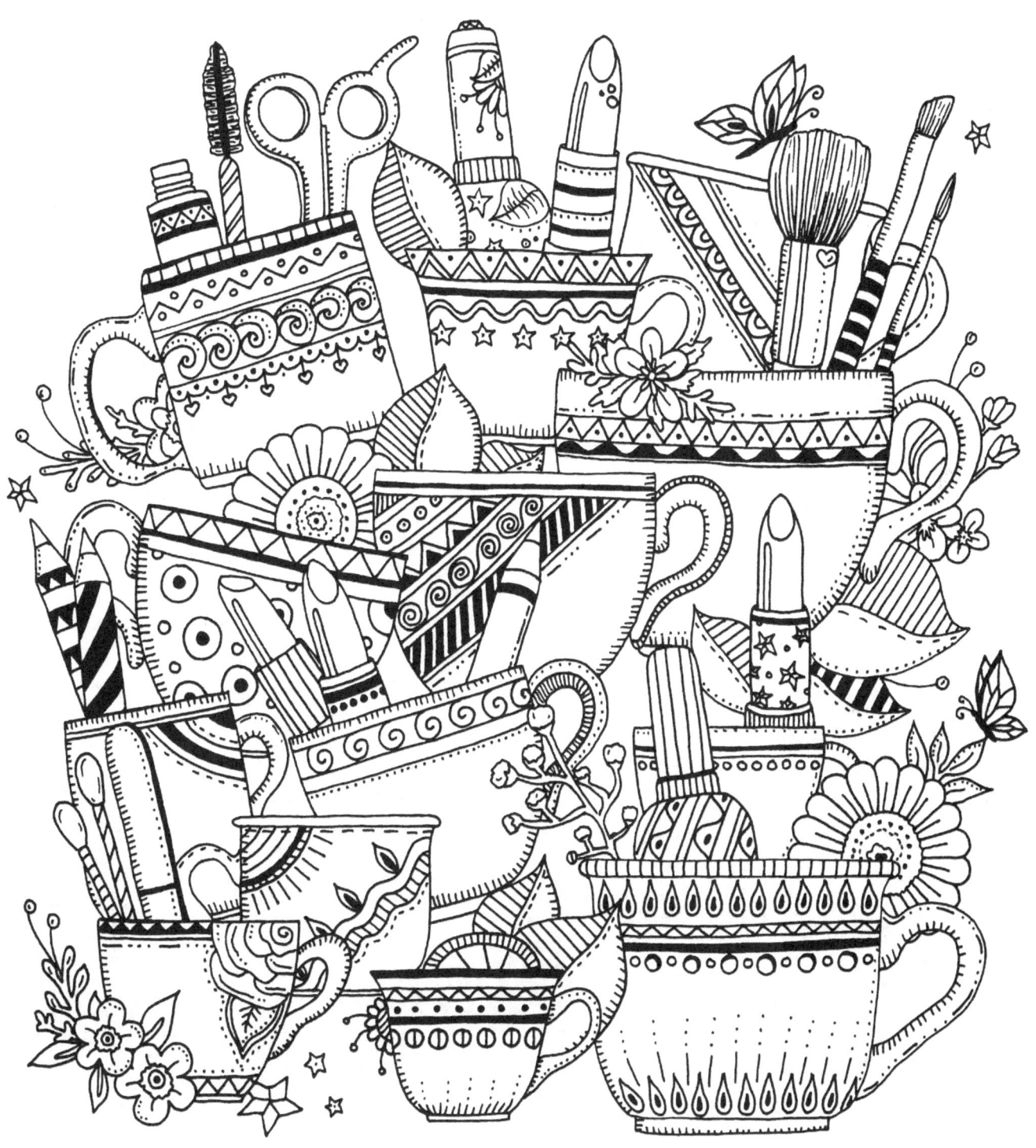

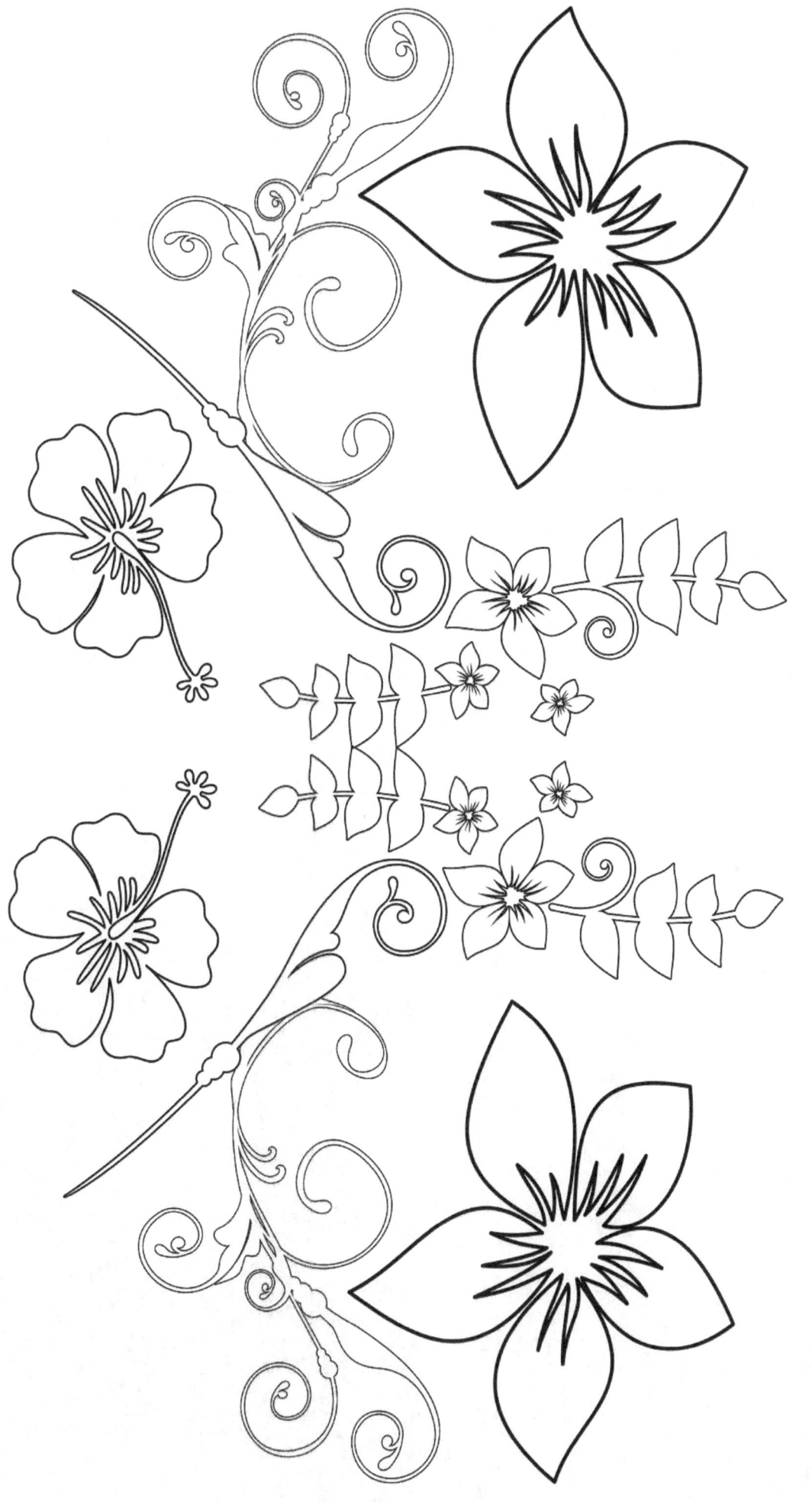

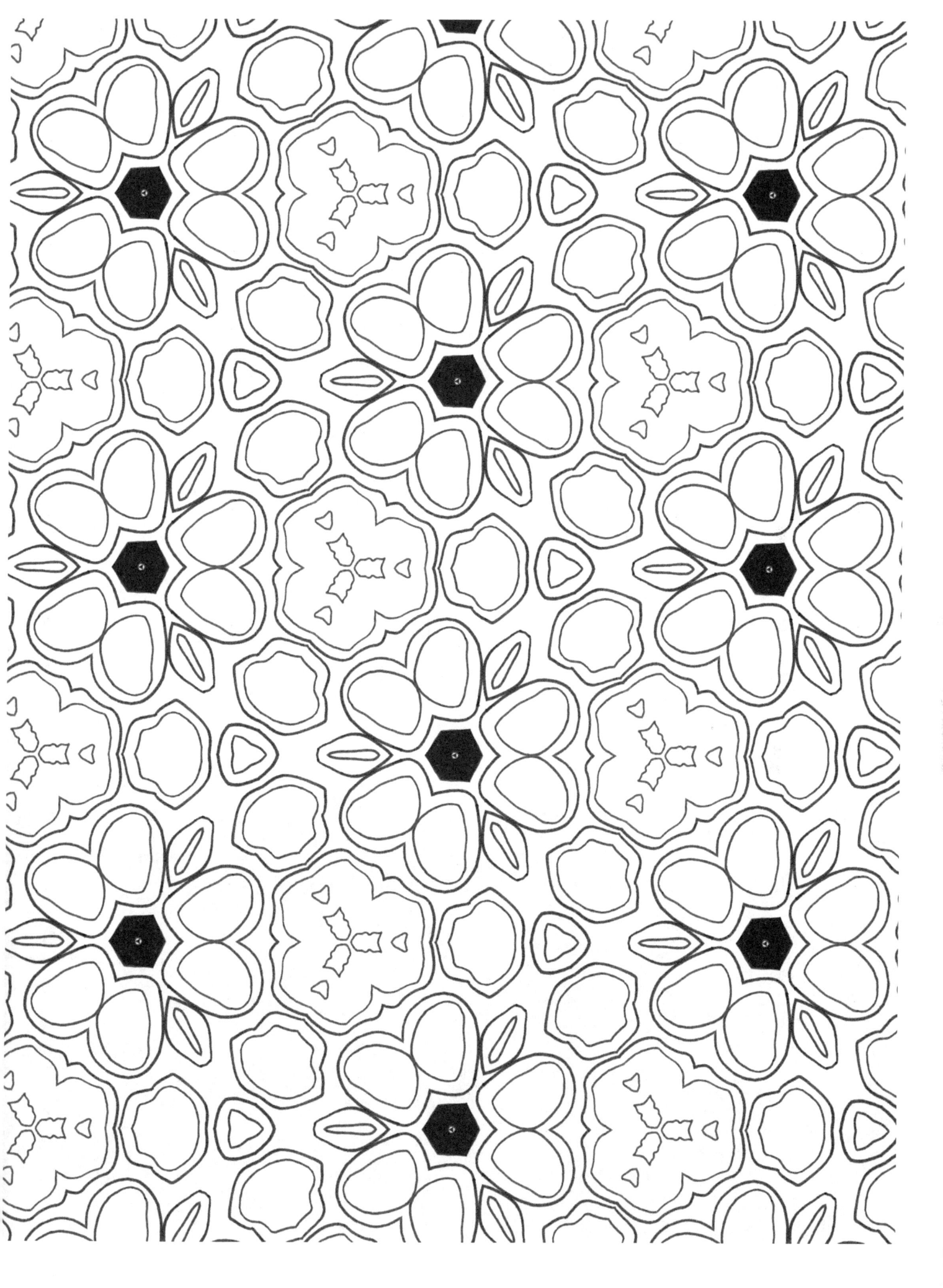

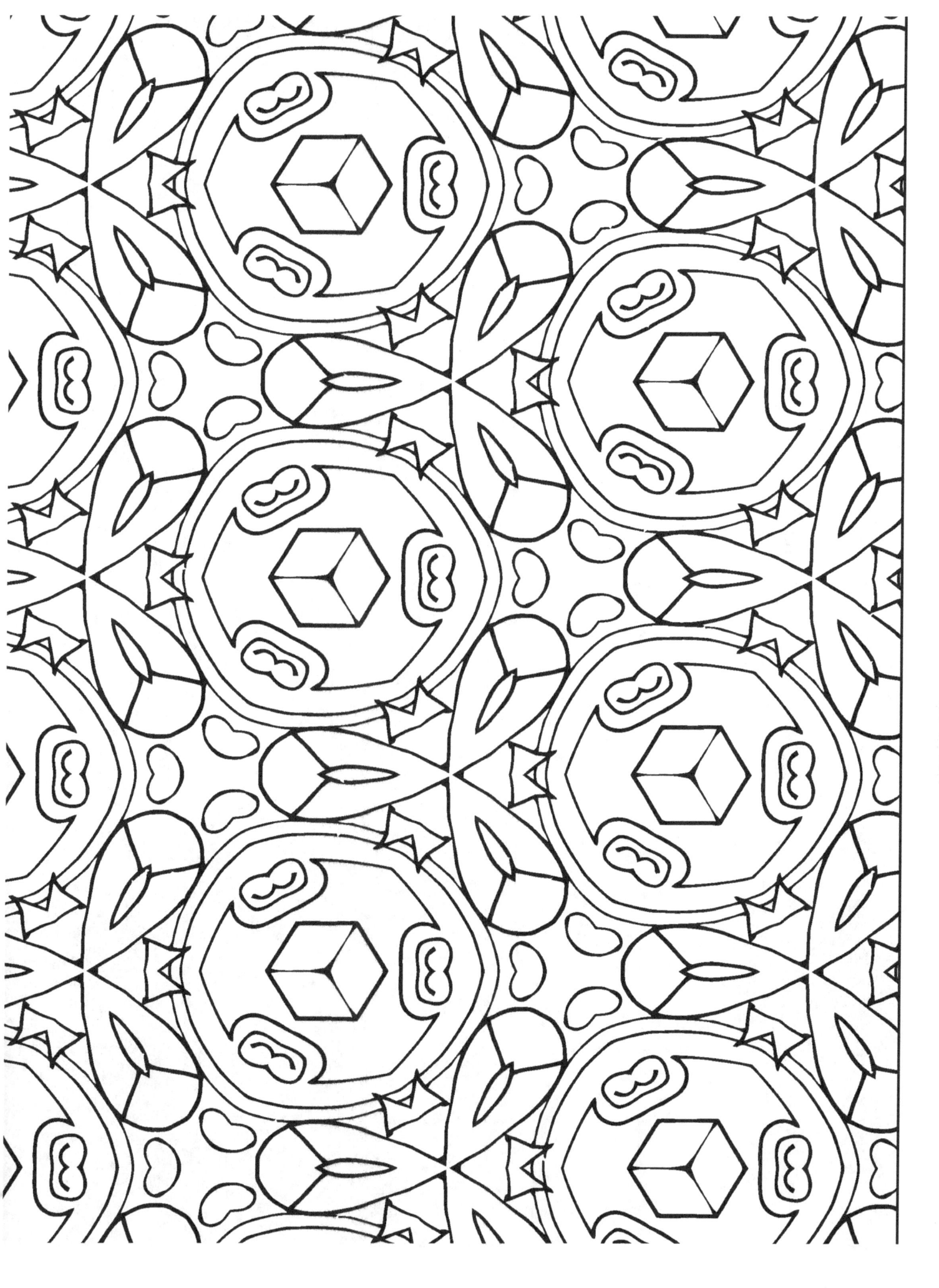

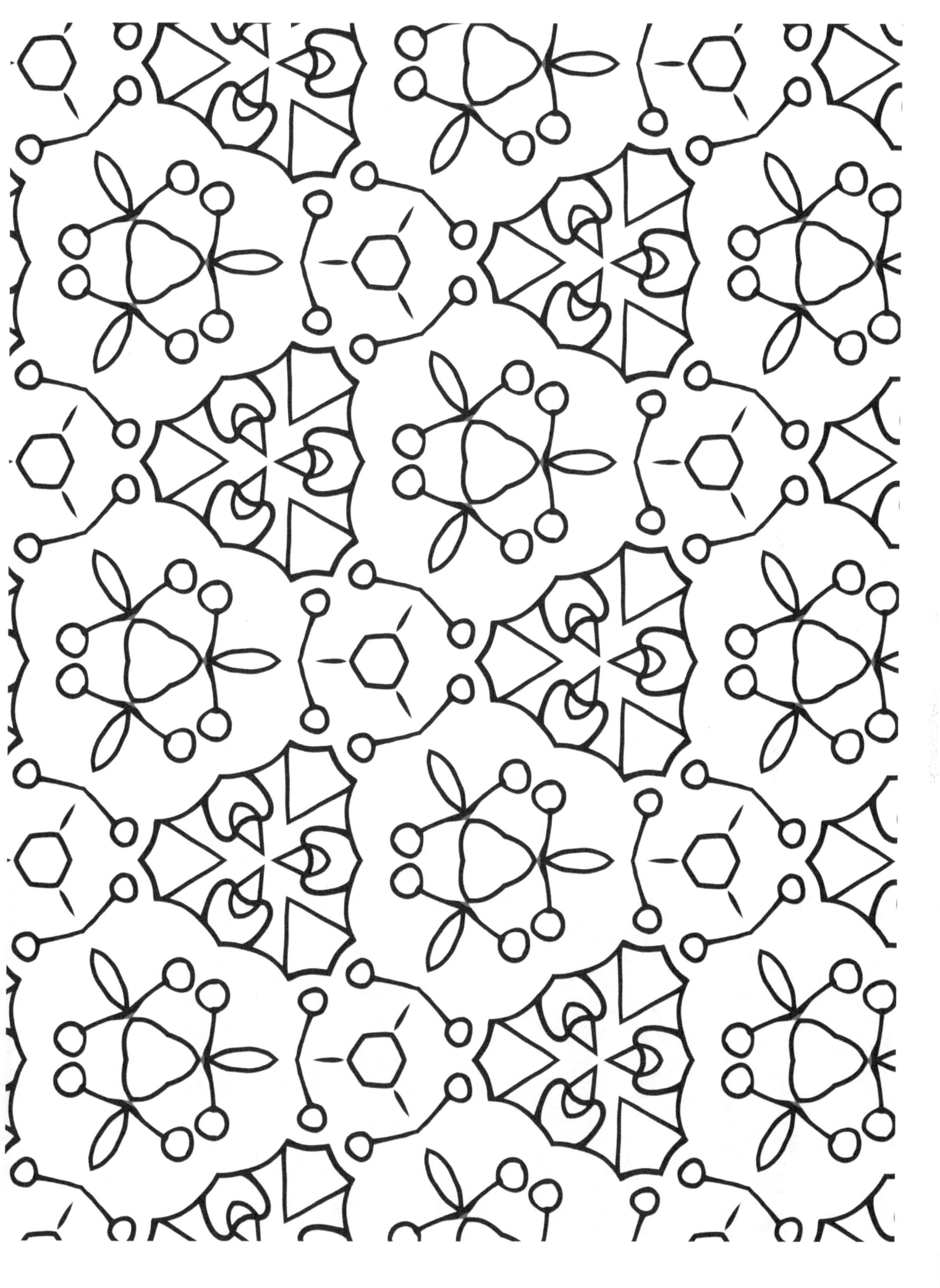

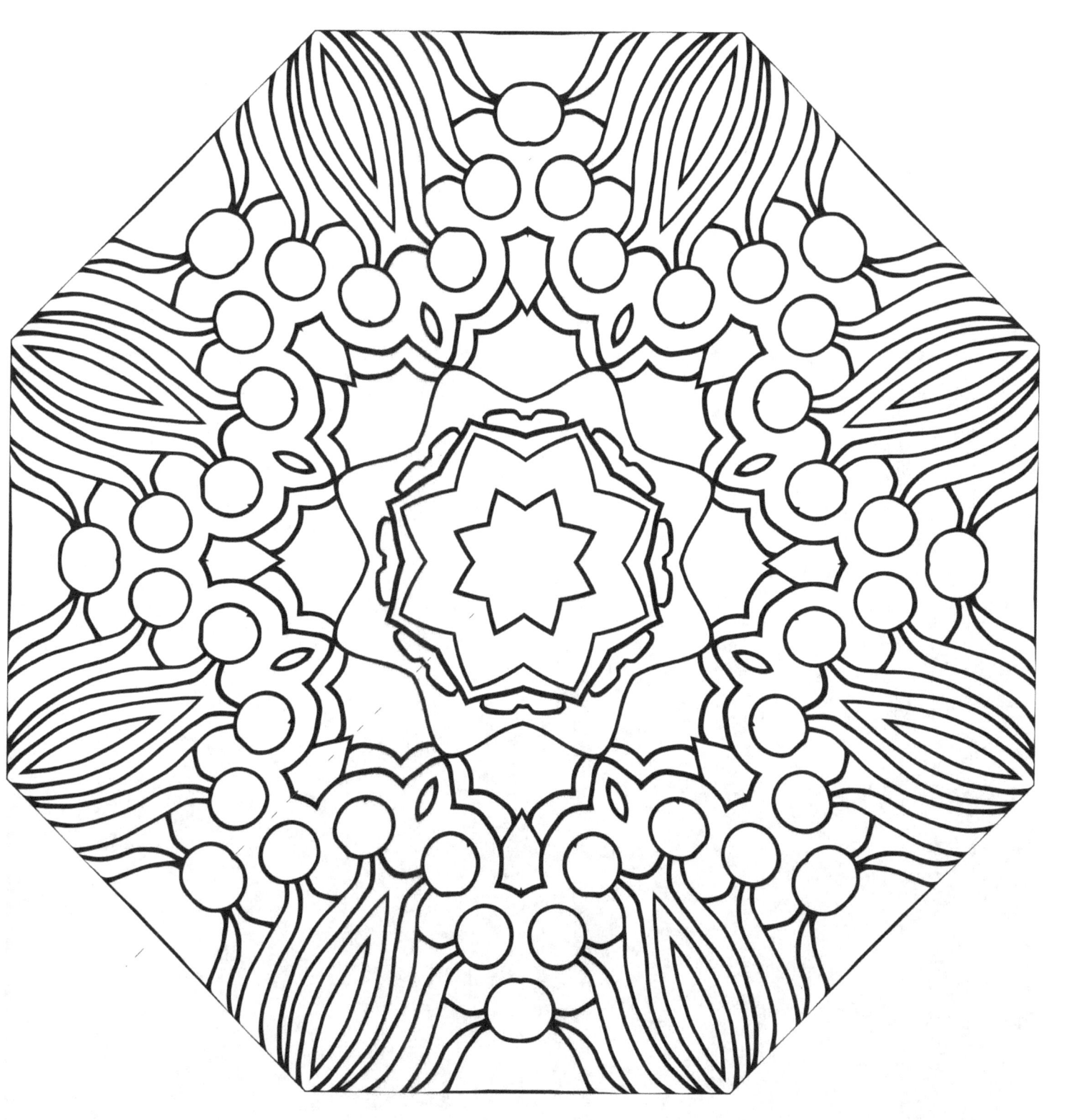

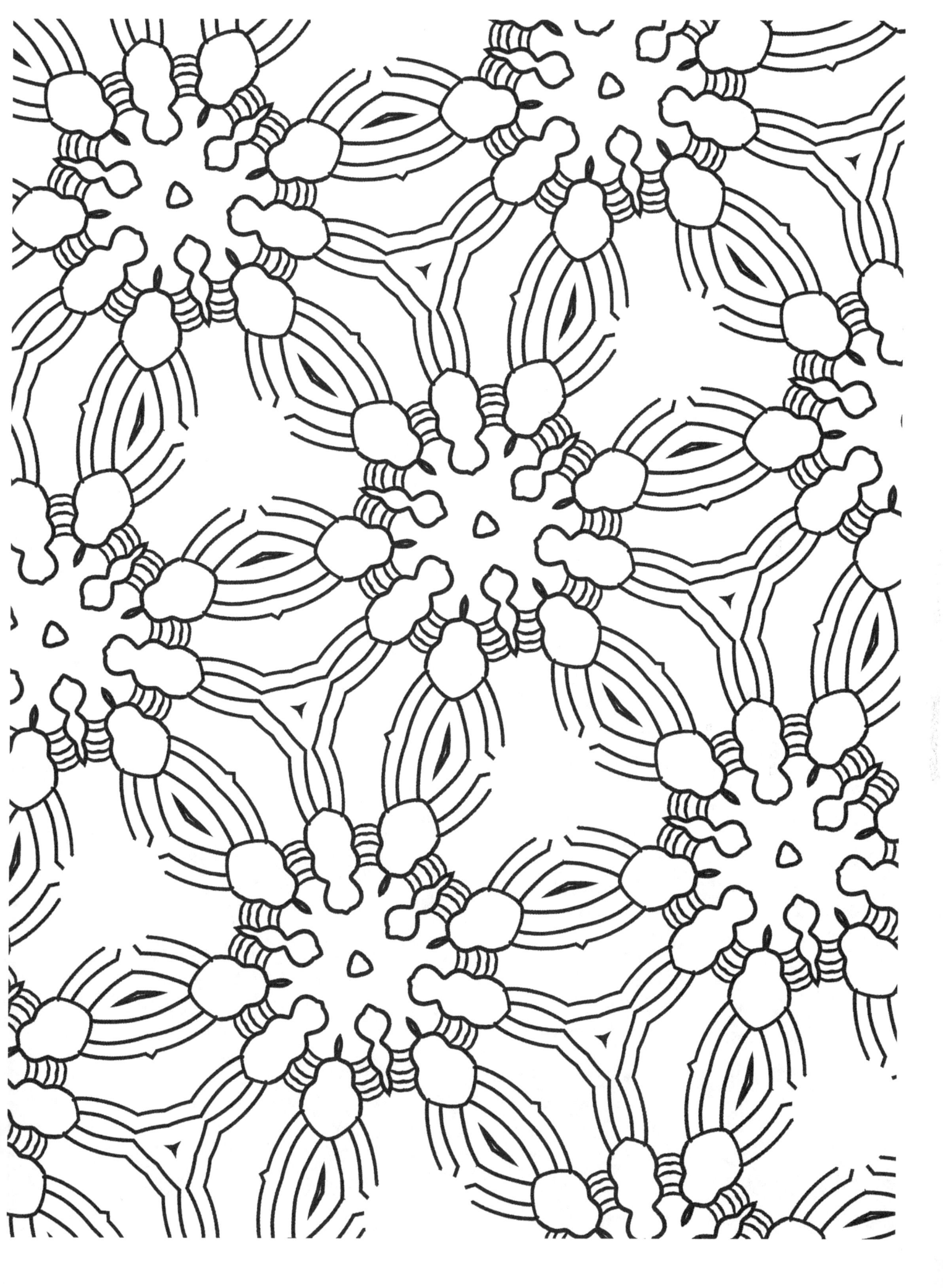

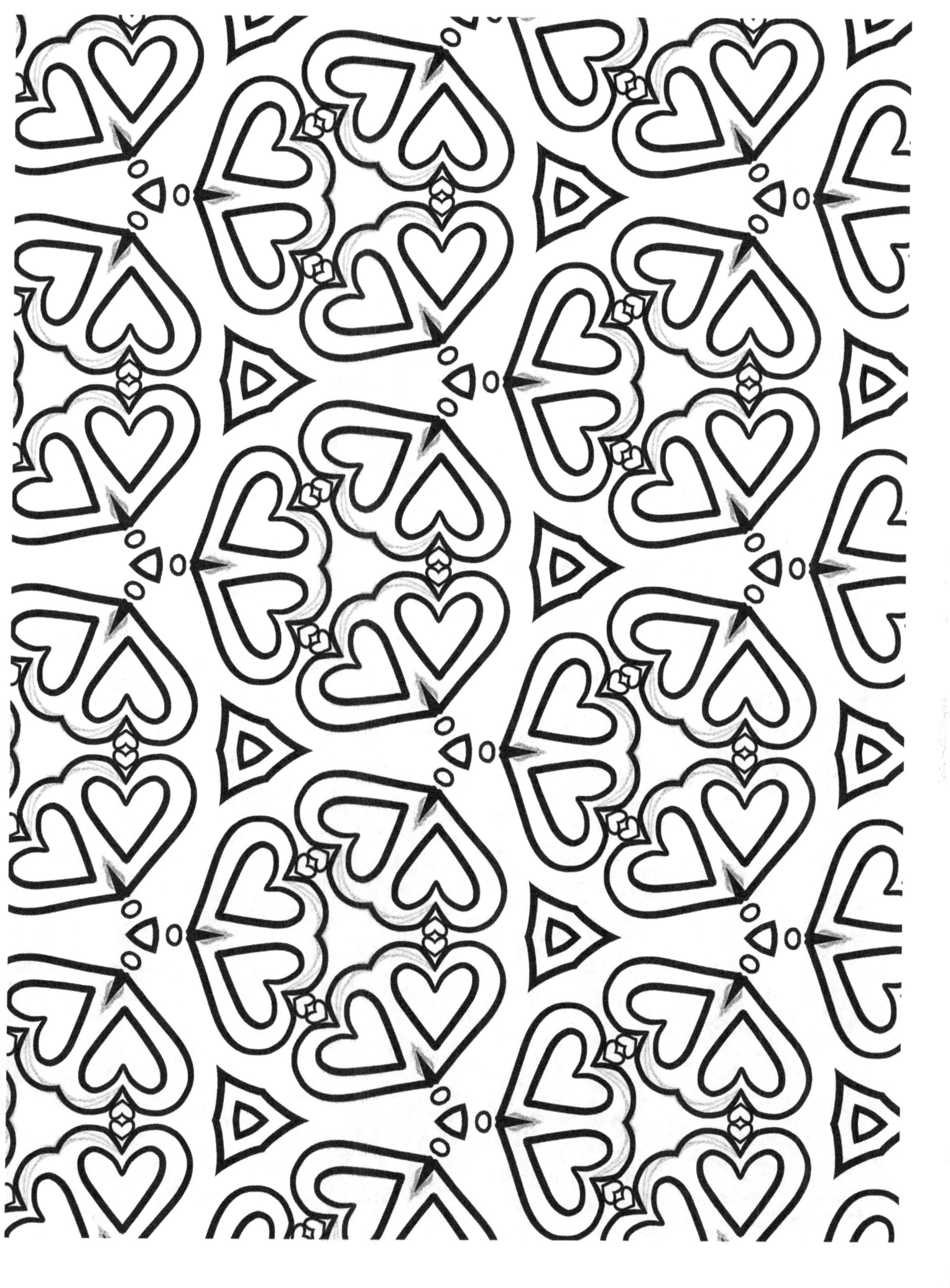

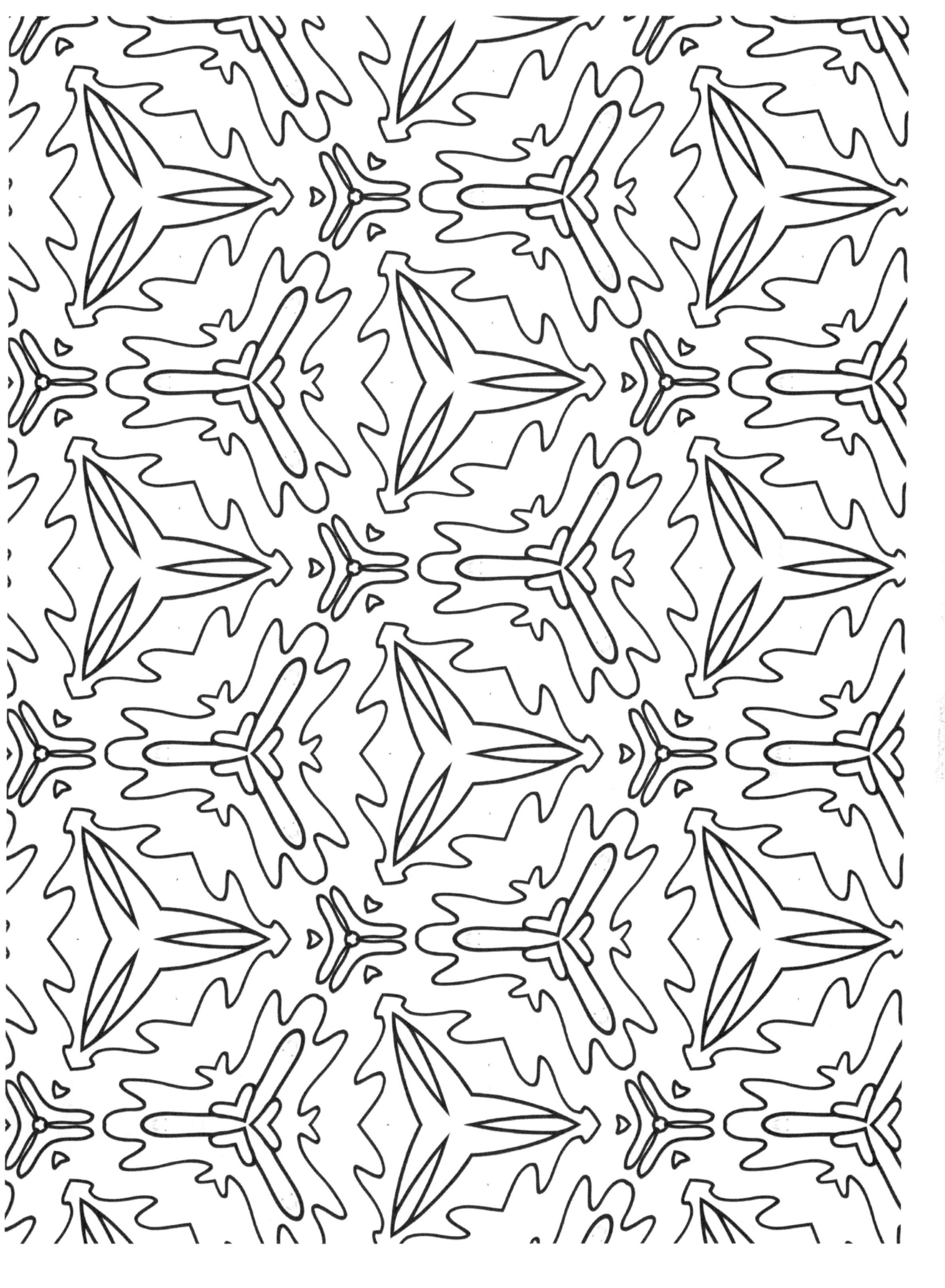

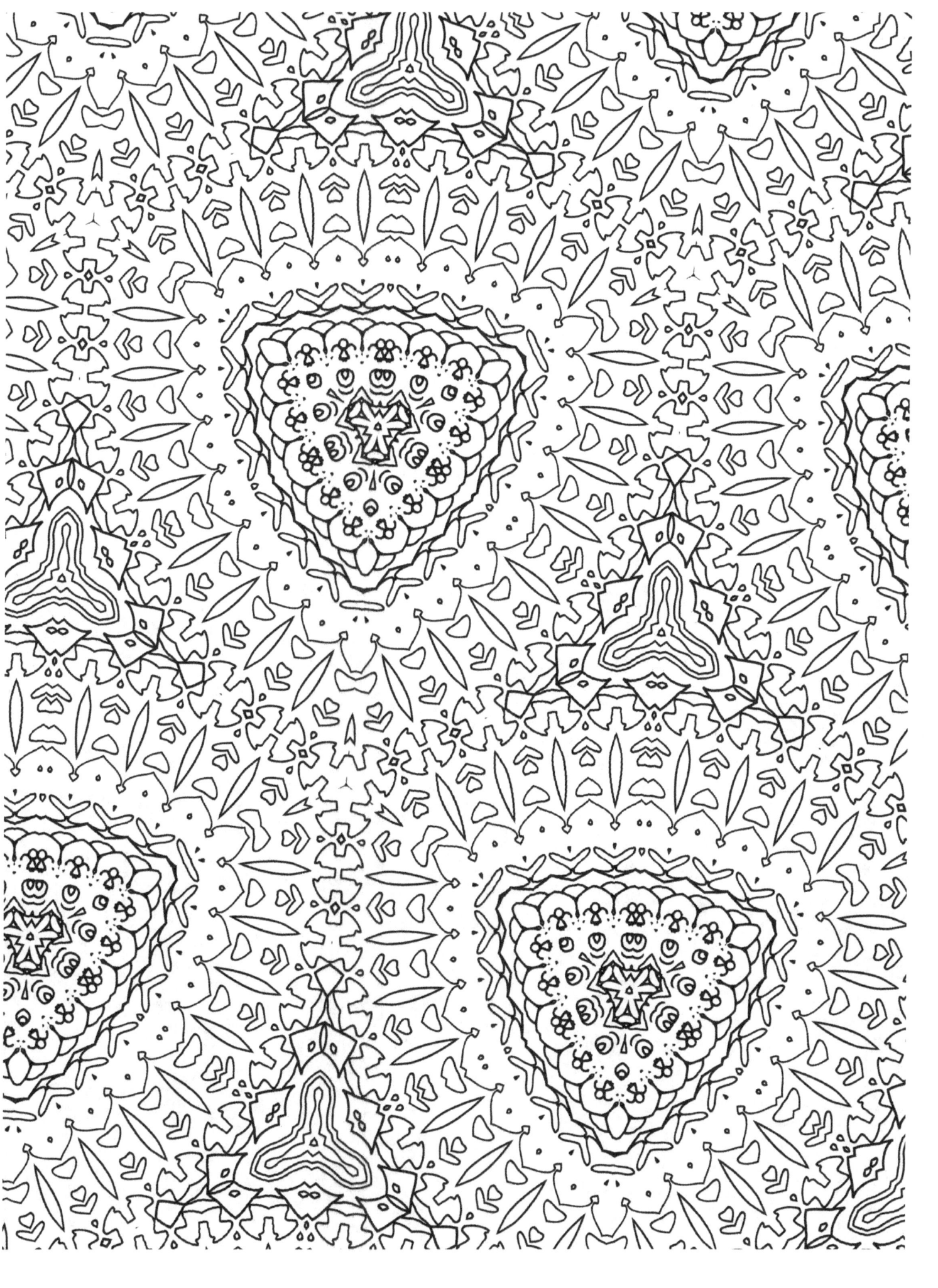

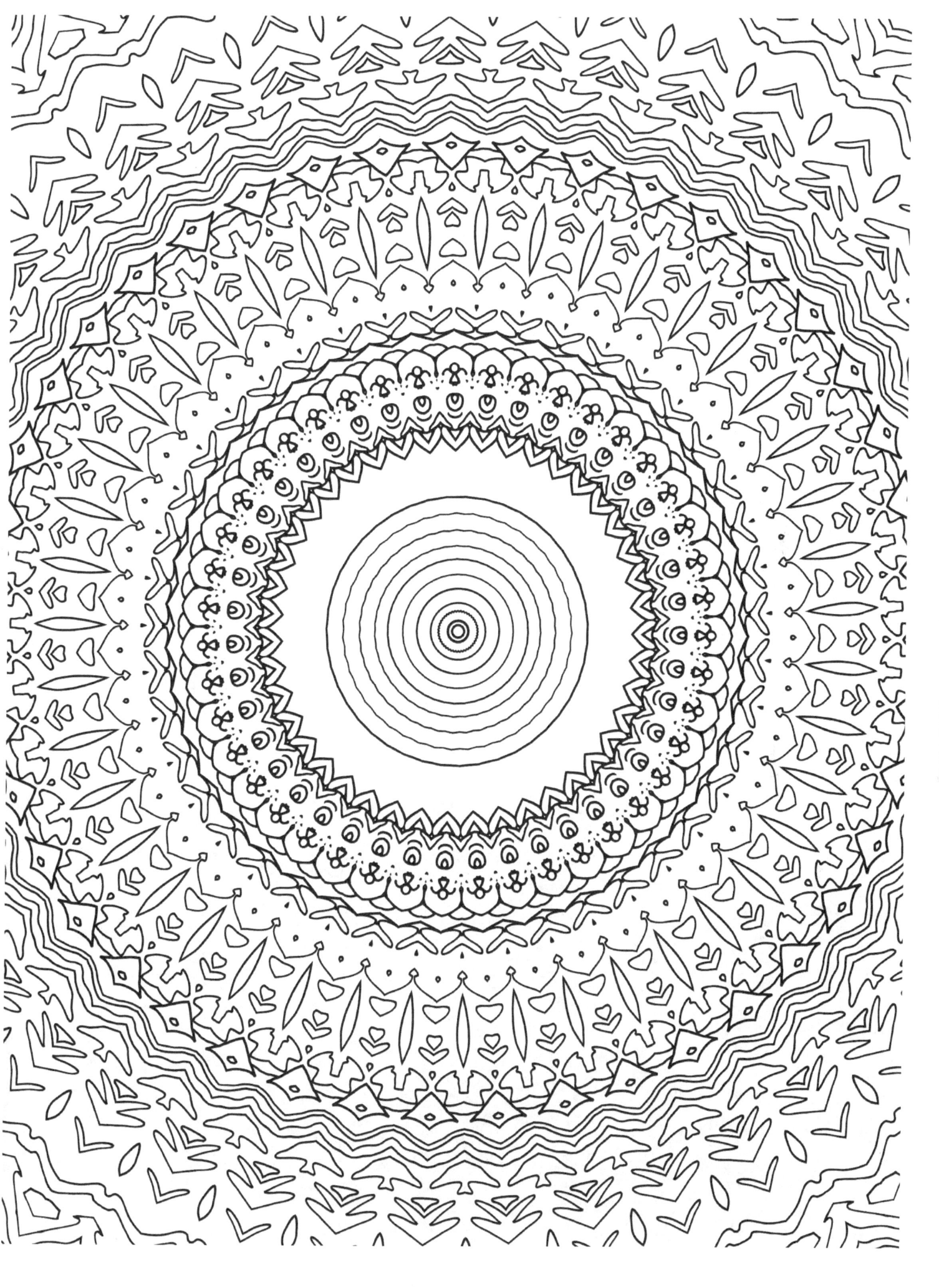

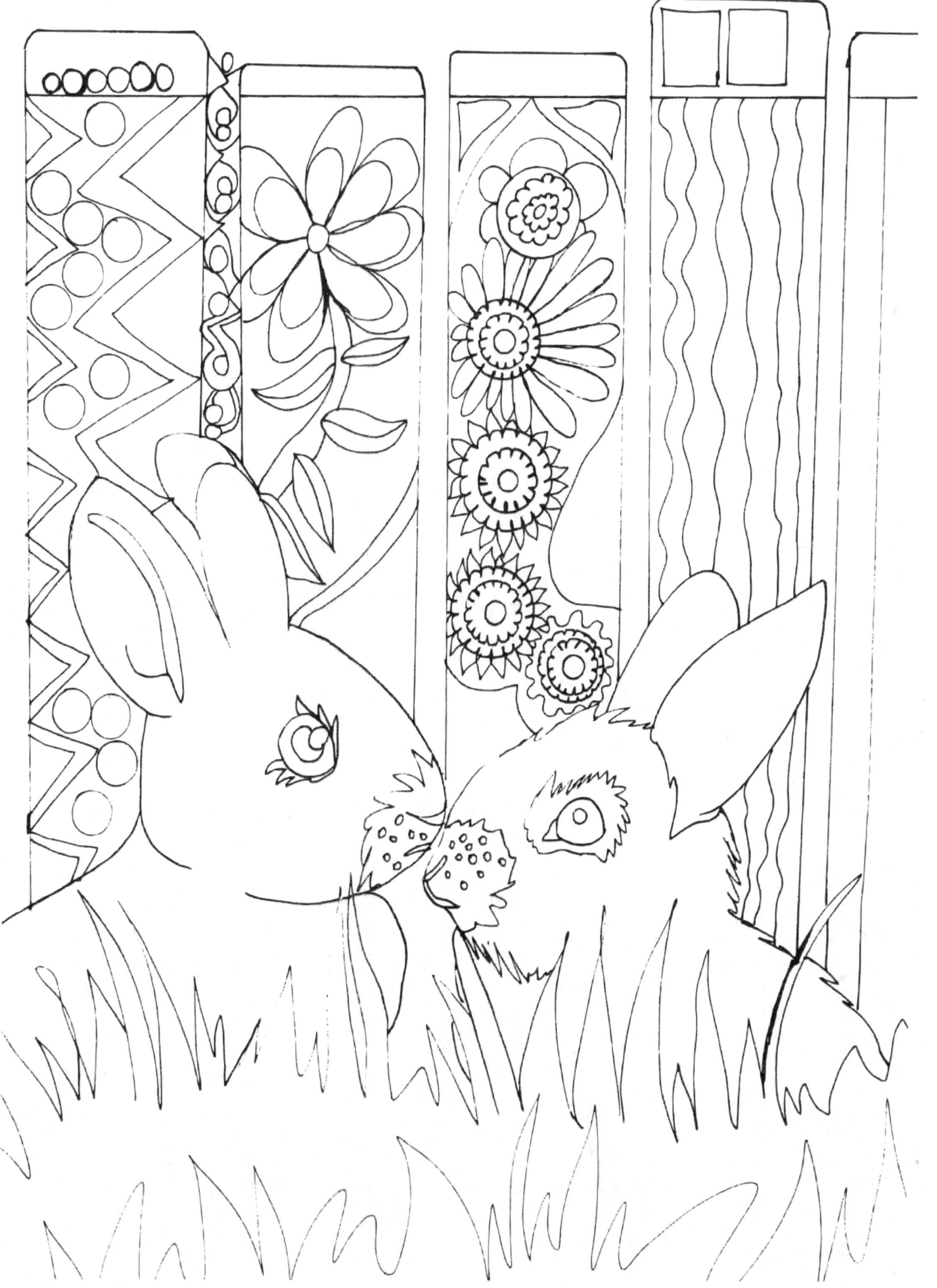

That's the end.

But let's keep coloring and painting to develop creativity and reduce stress.

Good luck!

Coloring Book
by: Samuel Lyons

Made in United States
Troutdale, OR
02/12/2025

28928706R00058